M000286258

Lord,
Get Your Needle–

I'm falling apart at the seams

The Emotional Strain of Chronic Pain

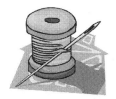

Barbara E. Haley

Chara Publishing House

Lord, Get Your Needle— I'm Falling Apart at the Seams

The Emotional Strain of Chronic Pain

Copyright © 2016 by Barbara E. Haley

Printed in the United States of America

ISBN 978-0-9975580-0-5

Scriptures taken from the HOLY BIBLE, NEW INTERNATIONAL VERSION. Copyright © 1973, 1978, 1984. International Bible Society. Used by permission of Zondervan Bible Publishers.

Quotes available publicly and taken from BrainyQuote.com, Christian-Quotes.org, Christian-quotes.ochristian.com, Christianquotes.info, Patheos.com.

DEDICATION

I dedicate this book to Gregory Len Haley, my precious husband of 37 years, who now resides in Heaven.

I smile when I remember how many times I called you at work to help me find just the right word.

I smile when I remember all the cups of hot chocolate and grilled cheese sandwiches you surprised me with late at night when I was in my office writing.

I smile when I remember a time I almost backed out of a writing conference because I didn't think I had what it took, and you said, "If you just spend time with Jesus under those majestic mountains, our money will be well spent!"

I smile when I think of seeing you again in glory. Thanks for your encouragement, your support, and your love, honey. I will always love you with all that is within me!

* * *

I would also like to thank Dale Schroeder, my Christian therapist and friend for many years. The first thing you taught me was how to put 2 Corinthians 10:5 into practice in my life. Your wise counsel, Christ-like compassion, and honest feedback has helped me grow in my understanding of who I am in Christ and all He desires to be in me. Thank you so much for allowing God to use you in my life, Dale.

Table of Contents

Introduction	**1**

Week One:

A Running Stitch of Hope	**4**
1.The Little Engine That Could	7
2. Hold On . . . I've Lost My Hope	10
3. Got a Piece of the Rock?	13
4. Great Expectations	16
5. Input. Output. Repeat as Often as Necessary.	19

Week 2:

Hemmed in with God's Presence	**22**
6. Why Can't Life Just Go Back to Normal?	25
7. A Secret Lesson	28
8. And the Verse Goes On	31
9. Let It Go	34
10. Now I Lay Me Down to Sleep	37

Week 3:

Cross-Stitched Love	**40**
11. How Wide . . . How Deep	43
12. No More, Lord.	46
13. And It Came to Pass	49
14. More Than Expected	52
15. Take Two	55

Week 4:

Invisible Stitch of Faith	**58**
16. Yes, No, or Maybe . . . I Still Believe	61
17. Has Anyone Seen the Lord Lately?	64
18. Have You Heard the Good News?	67
19. Time for a Lube Job	70
20. I Don't Believe in Suicide, But . . .	73

Week 5:

A Blind Stitch in the Dark 76

21. *Double Vision* 79
22. *A Starr Experience* 82
23. *A Few Notes About Peace* 85
24. *Feelings Object. Faith Answers* 88
25. *True Light* 91

Week 6:

Overcast Seam of Feelings 94

26 *Nobody Knows the Trouble I've Seen* 97
27. *The Truth About Lies* 100
28. *Lord, Take My Spinach and Give Me Your Spirit* 103
29. *Cross Check* 106
30. *The Problem with Peace* 109

Week 7:

Chain-Stitched Circle of Friendship 112

31. *Will the Real Me Ever Stand Up?* 115
32. *The Bottom is a Long Way Down. I Know … I Hit It.* 118
33. *My Bandage Isn't Sticking* 121
34. *What Do I Need?* 124
35. *Jesus Looked at Him and Loved Him* 127

. . . the Rest of the Story 130

Proclamation Scriptures

"Nothing in all creation is hidden from God's sight." Hebrews 4:13a

"You know when I sit and when I rise; You perceive my thoughts from afar. You discern my going out and my lying down; You are familiar with all my ways." Psalm 139:2-3

"Great is our Lord and mighty in power; His understanding has no limit." Psalm 147:5

"I have made you and I will carry you; I will sustain you and I will rescue you." Isaiah 46:4

"Therefore we do not lose heart. Though outwardly we are wasting away, yet inwardly we are being renewed day by day." 2 Corinthians 4:16

"[The Lord's] compassions are new every morning." Lamentations 3:23a

"We are hard pressed on every side, but not crushed; perplexed, but not in despair; persecuted, but not abandoned; struck down, but not destroyed." 2 Corinthians 4:8-9

"My God turns my darkness into light." Psalm 18:28b

"You hem me in behind and before, and you lay your hand upon me." Psalm 139: 5

"Know therefore that the Lord your God is God; He is the faithful God, keeping His covenant of love to a thousand generations of those who love Him and keep His commandments." Deuteronomy 7:9

"There is a time for everything." Ecclesiastes 3:1

"Faith comes from hearing the message, and the message is heard through the word about Christ." Romans 10:17

"Now faith is confidence in what we hope for and assurance about what we do not see." Hebrews 11:1

"Now to Him who is able to do immeasurably more than all we ask or imagine, according to His power that is at work within us, to Him be glory in the church and in Christ Jesus throughout all generations, for ever and ever!" Ephesians 3:20-21

"With man this is impossible, but with God all things are possible." Matthew 19:26

Proclamation of Hope

My hope is in God. His eye is always on me—nothing is hidden from His sight. He knows when I sit and when I stand, when I go out and when I come in. He understands what I am going through, for His understanding has no limit. God created me and will carry me, sustain me, and rescue me. I will not lose heart. Though my outward body may be wasting away, I am being inwardly renewed every day. God's compassions are new every morning. I may be hard pressed, but not crushed; struck down, but not destroyed. God will turn my darkness into light as He stays by my side, hemming me in—behind and before—with His presence.

My hope in God will not fail me because God is faithful and will keep His promises to me as I continue to love Him and keep His commands. This season in my life will someday pass—there is a time for everything. One day my tears will disappear and laughter will once again fill my days. Until then, I will strive to keep my eyes on God instead of my circumstances. I will continue to meditate on His promises because I know that my faith will grow as I listen to the Word of God, and that with faith, I can be sure of what I hope for and certain of what I do not see. Though I may not see the answers to prayer that I am looking for, I will hope in God, Who in His great power, can do immeasurably more than all I can ask or imagine. With God, all things are possible!

Introduction

Opening my Bible, I stared at the words. But my teary eyes refused to focus. "I can't do this anymore, Lord," I whispered, burying my face in the pillow. Outside the open window, a breeze blew and birds chattered in the trees. Neighborhood children laughed and played in their yard.

Gentle rays of soothing sunshine bathed the back of my body as I cried. But the comfort ended there. Inside, I remained untouched. Raw. Confused. For the very walls of protection I'd constructed over time to keep people out, also blocked the warm, healing light from entering my soul.

The constant, stabbing, abdominal pain I'd endured for months shot down my leg and worked its way up my side. I went from doctor to doctor. Maybe it was this. Maybe it was that. They tested, and I waited for the results, praying that perhaps this particular doctor might finally be able to determine what needed to be done to eliminate the pain.

Final diagnosis: pre-cancerous uterine cells, endometriosis and large cysts on both ovaries. Surgery, a complete pelvic reconstruction, took care of these problems. But complications left me unable to void completely without self-catheterization for a year. That led to muscle spasms and chronic bladder infections—at least one a month. At times I could barely stand.

I gave it my best, but my best came to an end. Sadness saturated my life. Controlling my emotions in public became almost impossible.

Truth often hurts. Like when we think about God's omnipotence. He is all-powerful. He can instantly change our circumstances and resolve our pain. The Gospels are full of examples where Jesus simply spoke a word and people were healed, the dead raised.

The Bible promises that the Jesus Christ of the Gospels is the same today and that He doesn't show favoritism. So why doesn't He heal us when we ask? How can we have faith that God will answer our prayers when we pray repeatedly and nothing happens?

As my pain persisted, I asked God these questions. Frightening questions. Maybe even irreverent. And God answered.

He cares. He loves us so much and wants us to bring our doubts and struggles to Him moment by moment. *Lord, Get Your Needle—I'm Falling Apart at the Seams* relays my experience. Questions and answers. Progress and setbacks. Life and death.

As I walked this path, I took notes. 2 Corinthians 1:3-4 tells us that God comforts us in all our troubles so that we can comfort those in any trouble with the comfort we ourselves receive from God. I wanted to remember the pain. I wanted to remember what I needed throughout my physical, mental, and emotional struggles so I could minister to others in the future. And I wanted to remember God's healing touch that penetrated my self-made walls and soothed my soul with peace and joy.

Helen Keller once said, "Character cannot be developed in ease and quiet. Only through experience of trial and suffering can the soul be strengthened, ambition inspired, and success achieved."

I pray that you will feel the warmth of God's arms around you as you work through these devotionals. That God will complete your healing in every way—physically, emotionally, spiritually, and mentally—and that as He does, you will realize how very much He loves you and wants you to come to Him.

At the end of each devotional you will find suggestions for personal journal writing. Please allow God to search your heart as you take time to meditate on His promises and write about your feelings and needs. Be still, and allow God to speak comfort, encouragement, and wisdom to you. He longs to fellowship with you, strengthen your soul, and fill you with genuine hope for your future.

"The Lord is near to all who call on Him, to all who call on Him in truth. He fulfills the desires of those who fear Him; He hears their cry and saves them."

Psalm 145:18-19

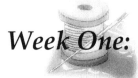

Week One:

A Running Stitch of Hope

"There is an eagle in me that wants to soar, and there is a hippopotamus in me that wants to wallow in the mud."

Carl Sandburg

Chronic pain touches every part of our lives. All day. Every day. Life becomes an emotional roller coaster.

We are exhausted. Sick of fighting the doubt and discouragement that accompanies our unanswered prayers for healing. Tired of feeling guilty for having no peace.

Our strength is gone, and yet we know God's Word commands us to be strong and take courage. But we don't know how to find the strength God is talking about. We can't fake it. The pressure of pain has crippled our faith, and we've learned to hide.

A world behind walls ... tolerable isolation. Emotional safety. We construct our refuge carefully, then burrow away—refusing to acknowledge or deal with issues buried deep within.

We shy away from family and friends, not sure we can trust them with our secret pain and heartache. We hide our feelings in private sanctuaries where only we know which key will unlock the door. A special song, a treasured picture, an intimate letter. Bridges to the memories and emotions now buried deep inside. Precious memories. Haunting memories. Memories held tightly, not to be shared.

Unfortunately, the walls we build inadvertently shut God out as well. When we see Him working in our lives, we open up and allow Him to bathe us in His love. But too often, when we can't decipher His plan, we incorrectly assume that He's not working, that He doesn't care, or that we can no longer trust Him.

The good news is that, even in times like these, we *can* have hope. Hope built not on circumstances or what we see and feel. Rather, this hope is built solely on the promises of God.

And this hope will not disappoint us. It is greater than we can even imagine. A totally new kind of hope straight from God, who declares, "As the heavens are higher than the earth, so are My ways higher than your ways and My thoughts than your thoughts" (Isaiah 55:9).

This week's studies introduce a hope that bursts through when we truly realize that we can do all things in God's strength. A hope that trumps circumstances and pain as we choose to accept the lifeline God throws us, climb out of the pit, and find shelter, safety, and security in His loving arms. (Okay . . . let's add *sanity*, too.)

This hope, more than mere desire, can withstand destructive powers. It is accompanied by expectation of obtainment and requires only that we continuously call to mind all that which God has promised us.

So, look up my dear friends. For "those who hope in the Lord will renew their strength. They will soar on wings like eagles; they will run and not grow weary, they will walk and not be faint" (Isaiah 40:31). This hope is available to you.

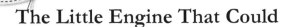

The Little Engine That Could

"The Christian life is not a constant high. I have my moments
of deep discouragement. I have to go to God in prayer with
tears in my eyes, and say, 'O God, forgive me,' or 'Help me.'"

Billy Graham

The phone rang, and I heard my husband answer. "She's
sleeping. Can she call you back?"

I rolled over and wiped my eyes. Time to shove the feelings
back down. Life had to go on. I couldn't sleep forever. "Oh,
God," I prayed. "Please forgive me for not doing this trial
right."

For months I'd waited as physicians ordered tests,
coordinated their schedules, and finally settled on a surgery
date.

It became tougher to pretend. To keep a smile on my face.
To maintain a joyful Christian witness.

During this time a friend invited me to a women's retreat. I
accepted, eager to spend time alone with the Lord.

On Saturday afternoon, several of us headed outdoors to
trample through wild brush along the Mississippi River and
savor the vibrant colors of the falling leaves and the pungent
smell of wood burning fires.

At one point, our path ascended the side of a steep rocky hill. I followed the others, but soon decided I hurt too badly to make it to the top. When I told my friends I was heading back down, they begged me to continue. "One step at a time," they pleaded. "You can do this."

So I continued. *I think I can . . . I think I can . . . I think I can.*

And to my surprise, after a few more steps, the path took a sharp turn to the left, and I found myself at the peak of the hill in a rustic scenic overlook.

As we fastened our jackets against the nippy fall air and drank in the breathtaking view below, we spontaneously broke into prayer and songs of praise and worship.

That memory carried me through many a dark night over the next few years as I endured one surgery after another. So often, when I felt I'd reached my limit, I remembered those last few difficult steps on that rocky hill and my friends' encouraging words, "One step at a time. You can do this."

Trials come and go—two simple words with a mountain in the middle. And the mountain is all we know for sure. Jagged rock looms before us. Fatigue and discouragement settle in, and life appears hopeless.

When we can do no more, we become still, and God is able to speak into our lives. *I know you can . . . I know you can . . . I know you can.*

Suddenly, a fresh burst of hope shoots through our soul. For God has promised that in His strength, we can do all things.

God understands our need to rest in the valley, to strengthen our spiritual muscles in a climb, and to be rejuvenated in His presence at the pinnacle.

So we continue, in God's strength, until He says we've gone far enough. Then the path will end—leaving us at a higher level than ever before. New challenges. New blessings. Closer to God. And ever so thankful we didn't give up.

"Let us run with perseverance the race marked out for us, fixing our eyes on Jesus, the pioneer and perfecter of faith."

Hebrews 12:1b-2a

Writing from the Heart
Healing ...from the Inside Out

How can focusing only on the steep, jagged rock in front of us bring us down mentally and emotionally?

What could we focus on instead? Be specific.

How could trusting that God's strength will sustain us to the top help make our climb easier?

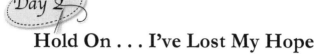

Hold On . . . I've Lost My Hope

"Get well cards have become so humorous that if you don't get sick you're missing half the fun."

Flip Wilson

God often uses humor to lighten our loads. Take doctor appointments for example. We arrive early, just to sit and wait. When our name is finally called, we sigh with relief—only to be led to a freezing exam room where we change into a skimpy gown and wait again.

Then there are the tests. At one point, my heart was acting up and I had to have a tilt-table test. The doctor explained that he would inject a drug to speed my heart up, and I would experience a rapid drop in blood pressure.

"This is a serious test," he said. "But I will be with you the entire time."

Right. Just as I began to feel a bit woozy, the doctor announced he was leaving. "Wait!" I said. "You promised to be here."

"I'm sorry, but I need to use the bathroom."

Not quite ready to let him go, I demanded an answer. "Is it a one or a two?"

As he hurried off, he called over his shoulder. "It's a three, and I'll hurry."

On a serious side, I've learned a lot about doctors. Or rather, about myself. Too often, I put my trust in a doctor, just to be disappointed when he couldn't help me. The doctors all agreed about what was wrong, but no one knew what to do.

It was after one of these visits that I wrote my thoughts.

> *A week ago Thursday, I went to a new specialist. I waited for the appointment for about three weeks. I thought, with all his credentials, he'd have some answers for me. I guess I had my hopes built way too high.*
>
> *The doctor was kind and thorough, but in the end, he couldn't help me. He referred me to yet another specialist. I walked out of the appointment with essentially nothing new. Extremely depressed.*

Hope is a difficult subject to write about. It's so personal, so revealing. Hope must be strong to survive, but almost never has any concrete support.

With hope, one can endure the most difficult of situations. Without it, life holds no meaning.

Hard to grasp, hope is even harder to sustain. Overwhelming rivers of discouragement and doubt—dirty waters pouring straight from the enemy—flow rampantly, forcing the small stream of hope to the bottom, hardly recognizable anymore.

The current seems so powerful, and yet, Isaiah 43:2 guarantees that when we pass through the waters, God will be with us; when we pass through the rivers, they will not sweep over us.

Turbulent waters will part as God's living water bubbles to the surface with a hope greater than all other powers of darkness combined. Hope that cannot be damaged, destroyed, or blown away by wind or rain.

Hope in God, based on His promise to never forsake us. Hope that ties us securely to God's lifeline as He guides us through storms and delivers us safely on the other side. Hope, and confidence, that there *is* another side ahead.

> "'For I know the plans I have for you,' declares the Lord, 'plans to prosper you and not to harm you, plans to give you hope and a future.'"
>
> Jeremiah 29:11

Writing from the Heart

Healing...from the Inside Out

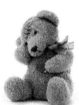

How could journaling about discouragement help us accept not being able to live a *normal* life because of health issues?

Talking about pain can relieve frustration and despair, but it can also breed negativity and bitterness. How can we control these results when sharing our burden with others?

God has promised that His grace is sufficient in our times of trial. What would that look like, practically, in your everyday life?

Day 3

Got a Piece of the Rock?

"Faith never knows where it is being led, but it loves and knows the One who is leading."

Oswald Chambers

Another doctor appointment—the whole nine yards. As women, we know the drill. Lie back, put your feet in the stirrups, scoot forward, and ... relax.

Relax? Who are they kidding? But thanks, Doc, for camouflaging those cold metal stirrups with brightly colored knitted covers. Oh, and the darling kitty-cat posters on the ceiling would alleviate anyone's anxiety, right?

Whatever. *Enough of the "homey" atmosphere. Just get finished so I can go home.* Then something funny happened.

The doctor finished the main exam and started a rectal exam, one hand busy checking out that area and the other pressing firmly on my abdomen. "Squeeze my finger," he ordered.

"How odd," I thought. His hand was between the thin paper sheet and my belly. "Does he want me to go under the paper or through it?"

"Squeeze my finger," he repeated.

"Oh, well. Here goes." With paper and all, I squeezed his finger as hard as I could.

He looked at me impatiently, and calmly said, "My other hand."

Talk about embarrassing. How did he keep from laughing? It was all I could do not to roll off the table. Somehow, I kept my composure as he proceeded to tickle my funny bone by suggesting I do daily rectal exercises. My mind would not behave. I kept picturing a group of ladies doing kegels while listening to "Sweating with the Oldies."

Funny story, but once again, this doctor was unable to "fix me." Once again, I battled thoughts that I would never be well again. Once again, despair settled into my spirit.

Proverbs 13:12 says that "hope deferred makes the heart sick, but a longing fulfilled is a tree of life."

My hope was gone. The word of the Lord was correct; my heart was sick. I was determined not to ask for healing again. It appeared obvious that God wanted me to suffer for some reason I would probably never be privileged to know. And I think I was okay with that. I believed in God's sovereignty— His perfect plan. I simply lost hope that I would ever walk in health again.

My life was battered and torn with the debris carried along in the mighty whirlwinds. I didn't know where to turn to search for hope.

Where was the living water? How could I hang on to hope when I had nothing left from which to draw strength? How long could I survive without hope?

Hypothetical questions? Not to those of us who deal with long-term pain.

Somehow, we must get ourselves out of the water if we hope to survive.

Will the current slow down in order for us to escape? Probably not. Chances are we might even have to risk a treacherous leap to get to a place of safety. A leap of faith to reach for a firm rock and cling to it with all we have in us.

Can we be sure the rock won't move when we grab for it?

Yes. Definitely yes. And as the waters continue to swirl around us, we can rest assured that we are secure in the Rock. Safe in His arms.

"Let us then approach the throne of grace with confidence,
so that we may receive mercy and find grace to help
us in our time of need."

Hebrews 4:16

Writing from the Heart
Healing...from the Inside Out

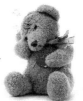

What does the phrase "Let go, and let God" mean to you, personally?

Why is it so difficult to actually let go and let God? Is there one area you would be willing to surrender today?

Write a letter to God explaining why it's so hard to reach out and trust Him, especially when you can't see Him doing anything. Be honest.

Day 4

Great Expectations

"Nothing paralyzes our lives like the attitude
that things can never change."

Warren Wiersbe

A few weeks before surgery, I heard a verse repeatedly—on the radio, in my devotional, in sermons, and in cards from friends.

"The Lord will never leave you nor forsake you" (Deuteronomy 31:8). What was the Lord telling me?

One day I joined several teachers who were sharing classroom tales. I smiled and pretended to have fun, but I felt isolated and emotionally distant. They didn't know the real me who rarely stopped hurting inside. Later, I wrote:

> It feels like my life is on hold. I have a hard time working. I hurt constantly. I can't make any future plans. It's just day-to-day living, just getting through.

> It hurts. It seems like no one understands the hell I'm living with. I don't want to be a bother to anyone, so I keep it all inside. But there's no way to get away from it.

Not knowing what to expect next is one of the toughest parts of living with chronic pain. Never being able to plan for tomorrow. Hoping we'll have a good day, but never knowing for sure.

We stop making plans with friends and family. It's embarrassing to repeatedly cancel at the last minute. Besides, spending time with others isn't what it used to be. We observe their carefree behavior and ache to be like them. We sink deeper into depression because we have no hope of life changing for us anytime soon.

Expectations. Let's dig deeper into this subject and how it relates to hope. According to the Merriam-Webster dictionary, an expectation is "a belief that something will happen or is likely to happen."

It makes sense, then, to carefully and deliberately choose our expectations. In some cases, this may help us avoid crippling frustration and heartache.

Further, we would be wise to *cushion* our expectations by choosing to respond instead of react if our expectations don't come to fruition. Pre-think the situation. Place our expectations in God's hands and remember that, ultimately, He knows what is best for each of us.

Finally, we must avoid *unrealistic expectations* by comparing that which we want to be true, to the reality of life. A great example of this is the tendency to think in terms of all-or-nothing. Huge red flag. An immediate setup for disappointment. Life almost never happens that way.

Now, let's look at the dictionary definition of *hope:* "to desire with expectation of obtainment."

We often consider hope to be a great desire for something. In regard to physical health, our prayers usually consist of desperate pleas for God to relieve pain and make us whole.

Our desire is tremendously strong, and as long as our goal seems possible, our hope soars. But when pain resurfaces, hope vanishes, and doubt, feelings of rejection, and anger immediately fill its void. Hope becomes a fleeting emotion.

But here is a new sort of hope that adds belief to our desire. A hope based on a sure thing . . . the promises of God. Totally believable. Every time.

"The eyes of the Lord are on those who fear Him, on those whose hope is in His unfailing love, to deliver them from death and keep them alive in famine. We wait in hope for the Lord; He is our help and our shield."

Psalm 33:18-20

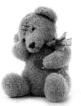

Writing from the Heart
Healing...from the Inside Out

Describe a situation in which you felt alone in the midst of a group of people. Why couldn't you connect with the others?

Name someone in the present or past who let you down. How has that affected your ability to trust others and/or God?

Some dreams or expectations only come to light when they frustrate or disappoint us. How could examining and becoming aware of what we expect help us develop genuine hope that won't let us down?

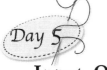

Input. Output. Repeat as Often as Necessary.

"Hope is the feeling that the feeling you
have isn't permanent."

Jean Kerr

Doctors agreed. Surgery was necessary. I looked forward to it—eager to have my problems resolved.

I checked into the hospital, slipped into my nightgown and settled in bed with a book. Shutting my eyes for just a moment, I relished the silence I so rarely got to enjoy as a first-grade teacher and mother of teens.

Unfortunately, my solitude was interrupted when a nurse appeared with a gallon of liquid. "I need you to drink a full glass of this every ten minutes to clean out your system," she announced.

No problem. I lifted the glass to my lips and took a large gulp. Immediately, my tongue curled in self-defense. I clamped my eyes shut and forced myself to swallow. The stuff tasted like metallic saltwater.

I tried to occupy my mind by reading during my ten-minute reprieves, but after several doses, I gave up.

You can do all things through Christ who gives you strength. The Holy Spirit brought Philippians 4:13 to my mind. I acknowledged my helplessness, God filled me with His strength, and I was able to continue.

Once again, I returned to my novel where the young heroine assured her fiancé, "God will never forsake us. He'll always be with us."

I smiled at the connection and thanked God for His reminder.

True hope, based solely on God and His promises, will never disappoint us. But there is a vast difference between *possessing hope* and *feeling hopeful*. Could there be a path from one to the other—even when pain and suffering torment us?

Actually, yes. The writer of Lamentations took such a path. One of many taken captive after the fall of Jerusalem, he described how affliction and bitterness depressed his soul. "Yet," he said, "this I call to mind, and therefore I have hope: because of the Lord's great love we are not consumed, for His compassions never fail."

Note the process. Input: *Yet, this I call to mind.* Output: *and therefore I have hope.*

What a great example of how to strategically redirect our discouraging thoughts to those that stir a spirit of thanksgiving and praise within us. How good to know that when we change our thoughts, our feelings will follow.

Perhaps this is why God's word instructs us in 1 Thessalonians 5:18 to give thanks in all circumstances. God knows the destructive power of despair and depression and the toll it takes on our spiritual, emotional, and physical beings. So He asks us to redirect our thoughts in order to find His healing peace.

Because of the Lord's great love, we are not consumed. Like silver refined in the furnace, we may be subjected to extreme heat . . . but never destroyed. Rather, our trials serve to purify and strengthen us. To make us more like Christ.

And when that truth really sinks in, and we daily *call it to mind,* hope will sprout. Discouragement will fade as we thank our God for His mercies and grace—new every morning.

> "And the God of all grace, who called you to
> His eternal glory in Christ, after you have suffered
> a little while, will Himself restore you and make
> you strong, firm and steadfast."
>
> 1 Peter 5:10

Writing from the Heart
Healing...from the Inside Out

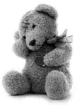

Which is harder to deal with—physical pain or feeling confused about God and His promises?

A Holocaust study revealed that the one factor common to all survivors was hope, or something to look forward to. How much hope do you have?

How can God's promise to eventually restore us help us endure our pain?

Week 2:

Hemmed in with God's Presence

"In these two things the greatness of man consists, to have
God so dwelling in us as to impart His character to us, and to
have Him so dwelling in us that we recognize His presence,
and know that we are His, and He is ours."

Frederick W. Robertson

Doctors do their best.

At one point, my blood pressure plummeted to zero when I
stood. For three days, I was stuck in the hospital bed while
the doctors sorted things out in my system.

Finally, the day came when I could stand. My first request: a
long, hot shower. But that didn't happen. I'd barely stepped
into the steaming water when a doctor arrived with a whole
team of interns.

"Mrs. Haley," he said. "Do you mind if I show these doctors
the inside of your nose? You have some very interesting cells
that I believe have led to your problem."

"Actually, Doctor, I'd rather you come back after I've dried
my hair."

The doctor turned in surprise. "I'm sorry, I don't have time to come back."

"It was a joke, Doc. Come on in."

Not that it matters, but that doctor was so short, he had to go all the way around the bed to see in the other side of my nose. I almost asked him if he'd like to borrow my overnight case to stand on. But I used my self-control.

As the team huddled around my bed, with a probe up my nostril and a light glaring in my eyes, it was all I could do not to say, "Boo!" when that little doctor got right in my face. I'm telling you, though, if I had it to do over again, I would do it. Wouldn't that be a scream?

Scream. That's what we feel like doing when we wait for days for test reports. One doctor said, "You need to stop thinking about this so much."

I really suspect that some doctors don't have a clue what we go through. We don't actually *choose* to think about the pain— we just can't get away from it. We go to sleep with it every night and wake up with it every morning. We spend hours alone with our pain, hiding from others because we don't want them to know our doubt and despair.

Alone? Not really. God promises never to leave us nor forsake us. Even in the times when we hurt so badly, we forget about His presence. Like a patient in a hospital room, too groggy to be aware we have a visitor nearby, ready to comfort and help.

This week, our lessons will remind us that God is always at our side, actively looking for ways to help us. To let us know we are not alone in our struggles. He will fight the giants. He waits with us through the storms and whispers His love in our ears.

As we soak up His presence, we find the strength to continue. The courage to trust Him with the unknown. The willingness to accept His perfect timing.

And as we learn to rest in His presence, our glad hearts will declare, "You make known to me the path of life; You will fill me with joy in Your presence" (Psalm 16:11).

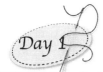

Why Can't Life Just Go Back to Normal?

"God heals and the doctor takes the fee."

Benjamin Franklin

Early the next morning, a technician arrived to take me to surgery. Startled, I argued that I was not scheduled until ten o'clock.

"Since you are having several operations, the surgery unit rescheduled you and prepared the operating room last night. I'm sorry, but we can't change the schedule at this point."

No one was with me, but after a phone call to my husband, the orderlies wheeled me to surgery. As I waited, I overheard my doctor scolding the staff. "Now there's no one here for her."

But I was doing fine. Fine, that is, until a nurse wheeled the bed ahead of me into an operating room. I realized I was next, and I panicked. Just as suddenly, though, I felt the presence of God and sensed Him saying, "Don't worry. I will not leave you nor forsake you. I am right here on this table with you. I am inside of you." A warm flowing sensation started at my head and crept down my body to my feet, literally bathing me in peace.

Deep in my heart, though, I longed for someone to hold my hand.

God heard my plea. When my doctor was discussing the mix-up, a friend of mine—another doctor—overheard the conversation and thought, "I know her. I can be here for her."

My eyes were shut, so I didn't see him coming. But at the exact moment that I cried out to God in my heart, this friend took my hand from under the blankets and whispered, "I'm here for you, Barb. I'll be praying."

I was never alone. God was there, just as He promised, ready to meet my needs—even before I asked.

Change is hard to accept. We have to adjust. Face tough challenges. Give up comfortable routines.

We can press on in God's strength or allow debilitating chains of bitterness and anger to defeat us and steal our joy and peace.

Perhaps we, like the Israelites on their journey to the Promised Land, become stuck in our distorted memories of how good life used to be. Or perhaps we don't really trust God to lead us into new territory. Too many giants. So we refuse and lose out on God's greatest blessings.

Or we move forward, believing God's promise in Isaiah 42:16 to "lead the blind by ways they have not known." He continues, "I will guide them; I will turn the darkness into light before them and make the rough places smooth. These are the things I will do; I will not forsake them."

God still works miracles today. In what area do you need God's touch? He is only a prayer away. He "fulfills the desires of those who fear Him; He hears their cry and saves them" (Psalm 145:19).

"These are the things I *will do*." I love that part. He doesn't say these are the things He's able to do or that He wants to do. No. These are the things He *will* do.

"You hem me in—behind and before;
You have laid Your hand upon me."

Psalm 139:5

Writing from the Heart
Healing...from the Inside Out

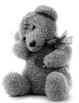

In what way is not knowing how you will feel from day to day like walking blindly through life? How can God's promise help?

Write about an experience in which you needed comfort, counsel, or encouragement to continue, and someone arrived at just the right time.

What about when you needed someone and no one came? How did you feel? Why didn't you try to contact someone?

Day 2

A Secret Lesson

"God cannot give us a happiness and peace apart from Himself, because it is not there. There is no such thing."

C.S. Lewis

I thought I knew pain. But the pain I'd experienced was mild compared to what I faced when I woke from my six-hour surgery. A voice mumbled through the fog, informing me that I was in recovery. Once again, the sweet presence of God physically washed over my body. *"I did not leave you nor forsake you,"* He whispered. *"I am still right here with you."*

"Barbara," a nurse called. "You need to open your eyes." I did as I was told and was tickled to discover that my nurse was the parent of one of my students and my technician was a guitar player in my church.

Not only did the Lord immediately reassure me of His presence after six hours of drug-induced sleep, He placed familiar people to care for me throughout the entire surgery. God's peace triumphed over fear and pain as God kept His promise in 2 Thessalonians 3:16. "Now may the Lord of peace Himself give you peace at all times and in every way."

Although I was heavily sedated for quite a few hours, the pain was intense as the drugs wore off and I began to wake up. At one point, a nurse asked, "On a scale from one to five, with five being the worst, where would you rate your pain?"

"Seven," I quickly responded. It was the worst pain I had ever experienced. As the nurse was leaving, she asked if I would like for her to turn on my music. When the soft praise songs began, I felt the peace of God, and my pain subsided. I relaxed and was able to rest. God was still with me. He was walking before me, preparing the way, and providing comfort for my soul.

At times, it feels like our lives have raced totally out of control. If this is God's plan for us, we don't like it. And *that* is exactly where we must start if we truly want to learn how to live with peace and joy in the midst of chronic pain.

God's plan. Can we trust it? Seriously, willingly, embrace it?

The apostle Paul lived daily with a physical "thorn in the flesh." And yet, he said, "I have learned the secret of being content in any and every situation, whether well fed or hungry, whether living in plenty or in want."

So what is this secret to contentment? Could it help us deal with our physical pain?

Paul knew he was not alone in his troubles. For he continued, "I can do all of this through Him who gives me strength." Paul continuously reminded himself that God was with him and would supply all his needs—physically, mentally, emotionally, and spiritually.

"The Lord will never leave us nor forsake us." We, too, can learn the secret of contentment as we remind ourselves of this promise, surrender to God's plan for our lives, and allow His strength to empower us and His peace to fill our hearts.

"Show me Your ways, O Lord, teach me Your paths; guide me in Your truth and teach me, for You are God my Savior, and my hope is in You all day long."

Psalm 25:4-5

Writing from the Heart
Healing...from the Inside Out

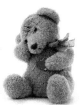

How could the process of *coming to the end of yourself* apply to your ability to accept your life with chronic pain?

Write about a tough experience in which you realized later that God was working behind the scenes on your behalf.

God chose to allow the thorn in the apostle Paul's flesh to remain. If God chooses the same for you, can you see yourself ever learning to be content in the grace and strength God promises to provide? What role would you play in learning this type of genuine contentment?

Day 3

And the Verse Goes On

"I would go to the deep a hundred times to cheer a downcast spirit. It is good for me to have been afflicted, that I might know how to speak a word in season to one that is weary."

Charles Spurgeon

My head throbbed throughout the night. I reached out in the dark to start my music. I had no idea what I had chosen, but as the music began, the soloist talked about the comfort God has to offer, saying, "Wherever you're at or whatever you're going through right now, God is there for you. He loves you, and He will never leave you nor forsake you. He is with you now and will be with you through it all."

Tears flowed as the song continued with those same reassuring words, over and over again. There was that verse again. And yet, it had become so much more than just "that verse." It had become God's touch in the dark valley through which I was traveling. Hope and peace and strength to help me overcome the hurdles I still had to face.

Why does God allow storms to cross our paths?

In 1 Kings 19:11-12, "The Lord said [to the prophet Elijah], 'Go out and stand on the mountain in the presence of the Lord, for the Lord is about to pass by.' Then a great and powerful wind tore the mountains apart and shattered the rocks before the Lord, but the Lord was not in the wind.

31

After the wind there was an earthquake, but the Lord was not in the earthquake. After the earthquake came a fire, but the Lord was not in the fire. And after the fire came a gentle whisper."

Elijah obeyed God, only to experience violent wind, an earthquake, and a fire. God was not in these storms. But afterward, God spoke to Elijah in a gentle whisper.

Could it be that God uses storms in our lives to capture our complete attention?

Need we be frightened of the storms? No. God is with us. Rather, we can sit them out as we joyfully wait for the Lord's gentle whisper. His intimate touch. That sweet, heavenly communion that can come only when we bow before Him and recognize His mighty presence and power.

When life shifts and we lose our footing, Christ is our only sure foundation. When storms surround us and mighty winds threaten all that we know, we must run to Him for shelter.

True, we may only be able to stay in God's presence a few moments before life's struggles yank us back to our circumstances. But each time we retreat to the safety of our foundation, we learn how to stay a bit longer. To focus on God even as unrelenting pain screams for our attention.

Practicing the presence of God. An exercise in self-discipline. Reminding ourselves to run to our Shelter when the storm gets ugly, rather than passively allowing the elements to wreak havoc on us.

Sunny skies . . . dark clouds approaching . . . storm in progress. Regardless, let's set the conditions aside and focus on God's love. Run to His waiting arms, for He will never leave us nor forsake us. In His presence we are safe.

"Call to Me and I will answer you and tell you great and unsearchable things you do not know."

Jeremiah 33:3

Writing from the Heart

Healing…from the Inside Out

Elijah was forced to wait through several storms to hear God's voice. Why do you think God's timetable is so different than what we would choose?

Life bombards us with busyness. How has your life with chronic pain slowed you down, benefiting you in terms of coming closer to God?

What changes could you make to protect and nurture your faith in times of trial?

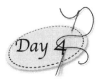

Day 4

Let It Go

"The truth is that the God of the Bible is the kind of God whose greatest delight comes not from making demands but from meeting needs."

Sam Storms

My body teemed with surgical gas the day after surgery, but since nerves around my bowel were still partially paralyzed, I was unable to pass anything. Nurses said there was nothing they could give me to ease the excruciating pressure on hundreds of internal stitches. The gas would pass in time.

When I cried out to God, an idea surfaced immediately. I should move from the bed to the toilet. A nurse helped me, promised to stay outside the door to my room, and cautioned me to push the alarm button if I had any problems.

As I sat there in extreme pain, nothing happened, and after a few minutes, I began to feel very weak and light-headed. Leaning against the wall for support, I pleaded with the Lord, reminding Him of His promise not to forsake me. "Surely You didn't give me this idea without intending to help me."

I considered giving up but thought about Christ dying on the cross for my salvation and for my healing. That thought led me to a song I knew, based on Romans 8:11. "And if the Spirit of Him who raised Jesus from the dead is living in you,

He who raised Christ from the dead will also give life to your mortal bodies through His Spirit, who lives in you."

So, with long pauses for strength, I quietly began to sing, "If that same Spirit . . . that raised Christ from the dead . . . dwells in me . . . dwells in me . . . He will quicken . . . my mortal body . . ."

And as suddenly as I mouthed the words, God did just that. He quickened my body and the gas was released. I laughed until I cried, praising the Lord for His faithfulness once again.

Looking back, I think about that pressure on my hidden stitches and realize that, too often, we harbor hidden feelings that cause emotional pain to radiate through our beings.

Anger. Rejection. Disappointment. Grief. Ugly, oozing infection that intensifies beneath tough scabs. Not gone. Just temporarily covered. Pushed away until new pressures in our lives cause it to flare again. Pressures we cannot control.

As we sit in the bathrooms of life, waiting on God's response, we might be tempted to give up. To reason that God's touch is not meant for us at this time. But even at our lowest point, let's remember that the same Spirit who raised Christ from the dead lives in us.

His presence dwells within our hearts to change our lives. Quickens our mortal bodies. Shakes us up enough to reveal that which needs to be acknowledged and cleansed. God not only wants to heal our physical bodies; He is interested in our souls—our mind, will, and emotions.

In His presence, as we surrender our feelings and fears, He will treat our wounds and facilitate inner healing. Because only then, will the pain be gone for good.

> "I will give you a new heart and put a new spirit in you;
> I will remove from you your heart of stone and
> give you a heart of flesh."
>
> Ezekiel 36:26

Writing from the Heart

Healing…from the Inside Out

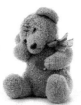

What feelings, thoughts, and issues in your life would you rather not face?

Do they nag at you constantly or just pop up unexpectedly at random times? Can you identify triggers that cause them to surface?

What effect do you think this emotional baggage has on your physical condition?

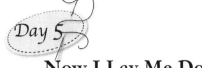

Now I Lay Me Down to Sleep

"We may ignore, but we can nowhere evade, the presence of God. Though our feelings come and go, God's love for us does not."

C.S. Lewis

Sleep evaded me for two days. I stared blankly at the ceiling—unable to relax. My head ached and my heart raced, sporadically skipping beats. At night, ghoulish figures slithered around the ceiling and walls of my room. No matter how hard I tried, I couldn't blink them away.

David's cry from Psalm 6:3,6 became mine. "My soul is in deep anguish. How long, Lord, how long? . . . I am worn out from my groaning. All night long I flood my bed with weeping and drench my couch with tears."

I'd known God for thirty-five years, but I'd never walked through such a difficult trial. I'd never been so weak that I wondered if I would even survive. I'd never actually questioned God's presence in my life.

When my doctor made his rounds the next morning, I told him about the hallucinations. He smiled with understanding. "You're suffering from sleep deprivation. I need to get you home where you will be more comfortable. You'll be able to sleep there."

As he talked to me about caring for myself, he explained that he was going to change one of my prescriptions to something that had medicine in it for my headaches. "It will actually be better for you because the drug you have been taking has quite a bit of caffeine in it."

BINGO! I've always reacted negatively to caffeine—it gives me severe headaches and heart palpitations. I had no idea medicine could contain caffeine. But God, in His goodness, allowed the error to be discovered before I left the hospital.

Sleep deprivation alters our perspective, our moods, and our memories. Charles Stanley points out that we often fail to remember former answers to prayer, times when the Holy Spirit has guided us, and previous lessons we've learned. He adds, "Only the present seems real. Our minds spin with future implications, and our troubled emotions inhibit clear thinking."

Satan knows our vulnerability in such times of weakness and pounces on the opportunity to convince us to stop praying. Stop seeking. Stop hoping.

But as we remain in God's presence, He will protect us.

Hosea 2:14-15 speaks of God's desire to gently work in us, to bring good from our pain, and to restore the joy of our salvation. "Therefore I am now going to allure her; I will lead her into the desert and speak tenderly to her. There I will give her back her vineyards, and will make the Valley of Achor a door of hope. There she will sing as in the days of her youth, as in the day she came up out of Egypt."

Achor means trouble. God has called us to Himself and will make our valley of trouble a door of hope. He has led us into a type of desert, away from distraction and temptation, so He might speak tenderly to our spirits. He will free us from those things that hold us captive, give us rest, and restore our joy.

"So do not fear, for I am with you; do not be dismayed, for I am your God. I will strengthen you and help you; I will uphold you with My righteous right hand."

Isaiah 41:10

Writing from the Heart
Healing...from the Inside Out

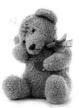

How does life become more difficult when you are not rested?

When life overwhelms us, Satan often whispers words of condemnation into our ears. How could memorizing Scripture and listening to Christian music help ward off the enemy?

What personal heartache or pain are you carrying that you don't want anyone but God to know about? Take time to write to God about it and let Him comfort you.

Week 3:

Cross-Stitched Love

"God proved His love on the cross. When Christ hung, and bled, and died, it was God saying to the world, 'I love you.'"

Billy Graham

One day, as I held my infant granddaughter in my arms and fed her a bottle, she looked intently into my eyes and reached up with her little fingers to touch my cheek. Words can't describe the powerful bolt of love that surged through my heart. I never wanted to let the sweet thing go.

That night, when I woke in pain, I asked the Lord to remind me that He was still with me. The picture of the baby in my arms immediately came to mind, and the Lord said, "You remember the deep love you felt for the baby? I love you *that* much . . . and much, much more."

Ooh. How good it would be to be a child again. Unaware of the confusing complexities of life. Unconcerned with distressing decisions. Unburdened with self-imposed proprieties.

Precious memories for some. But in reality, many of us did not enjoy a loving childhood or a nurturing relationship with our earthly fathers. Or maybe we did, but at some point, he abandoned us or let us down. And so . . . our concept of father-love was formed.

Life, as an adult, is difficult. Being strong is exhausting. Unlike a child, we no longer have a parent to whom we can bring our questions, heartaches, bumps and bruises. No one to run to for shelter when the storms get too rough.

Or do we? Luke 18:17 states that "Anyone who will not receive the kingdom of God like a little child will never enter it." God sees the frightened child in us. He realizes we need to learn to let go and allow ourselves to come to Him with our deepest feelings and needs. To know His love, relax in His care, and trust Him as Father.

God's love and favor have absolutely nothing to do with performance. Rather, like the tiny child I held in my arms, God loves us just because we are His children.

In this week's lessons, we'll drill down into our belief systems to uncover the depths of God's great love for us. We'll discover that God sometimes allows trials in our lives to teach us just how much He loves us. That He will never leave us nor forsake us. That as we run to Him, He runs to us.

We will consider Christ as our Great Physician who knows exactly how to mend us. Our eyes will be opened as we realize God is personally involved in our care, even when circumstances seem to say otherwise. That He is busy pruning and shaping us into His image, for our good and His glory.

We'll be introduced to a Father-love that is complete in every way. One that knows our every need, carries our heavy burdens, and sets us free. Free to frolic in His love and grace as a child, yet strong enough to faithfully walk the path He sets before us. Supernatural, unconditional, unlimited love. For that is who God is.

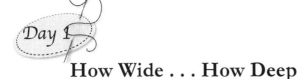

How Wide . . . How Deep

"Snuggle in God's arms. When you are hurting, when you feel lonely, left out. Let Him cradle you, comfort you, reassure you of His all-sufficient power and love."

Kay Arthur

The morning finally came for me to go home. I was weak and unable to eat. All I wanted was to go home and get into my own bed. Some friends stopped by as I waited for the nurse to bring the discharge papers. They apologized for not coming sooner, but God knew when they needed to be there.

While we were talking, a nurse came in. "Excuse me, folks," she said. "Mrs. Haley, your last urine test showed a large amount of bacteria, so your doctor has ordered a major shot of antibiotics. It will be quite painful, so he ordered this pill to help you relax. Here you go." I took the pill and swallowed a drink of water. "I'll be back in about five minutes," the nurse said as she disappeared in the hallway.

As soon as she left, I broke. My friend held me while her husband prayed. I don't know what I would have done if they had not been there. God sent them at just the right moment to minister to me when I could take no more.

The nurse returned shortly to give me the shot. I shut my eyes, waiting. After a moment, I asked, "How long will you have to leave the needle in?"

Astonished, she exclaimed, "What do you mean? I'm already finished. Surely you felt that."

"No," I cried. "We just prayed, and God took that one for me." In a small way, the experience reminded me of the cross on which Christ suffered for my transgressions.

As I recovered, I often asked why God allowed me to suffer such pain. Why He didn't heal me instantly when I first prayed for healing.

I believe it was all for a child who needed to learn just how much her Father loved her. To know, beyond any doubt, that He would never leave her nor forsake her. That even in the midst of pain and suffering, He would be there.

God's word is true. He was with me before surgery—giving me grace and strength to endure the pain. He was with me during surgery—staying close by to protect me. And He was with me throughout my recovery—meeting all my needs before I even asked.

Nothing is hidden from God. He's aware of the path of pain and despair we are on—every sharp turn, every steep hill. Nothing passes unseen before His eyes.

Oh, what comfort to know that we never need to be afraid. That God will always be with us. In times of joy or sorrow, in times of strength or weakness.

James 4:8 says, "Come near to God and He will come near to you." I used to picture Him waiting with open arms as I ran to Him. But that's not what the verse says. Rather, as we run to God, He *runs* to us. His arms opened wide, He's anxious to embrace us as soon as possible. That's the kind of Father-love He has for us!

"And I pray that you, being rooted and established in love, may have power, together with all the Lord's holy people, to grasp how wide and long and high and deep is the love of Christ, and to know this love that surpasses knowledge—that you may be filled to the measure of all the fullness of God."

Ephesians 3:17-19

Writing from the Heart
Healing...from the Inside Out

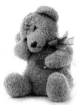

Write about a time when God showed you His love through other people.

How has your earthly father's love, or lack thereof, influenced your concept of God's Fatherly love?

How has God used uncomfortable circumstances in your life to reveal the depths of His Father-love?

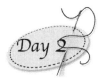

No More, Lord.

"Your most profound and intimate experiences of worship
will likely be in your darkest days—when your heart is
broken, when you feel abandoned, when you're out of
options, when the pain is great—and you turn to God alone."

Rick Warren

Once I got home from the hospital, I became weaker and
weaker. I tried to eat, but even the tiniest piece of a cracker
caused me to heave. At that point, I didn't care anymore. I
really didn't think I was going to make it.

As my children left for school, I honestly thought I would
never see them again. I held them tightly, told them I loved
them and asked them to pray for me before they left.

Looking back, I see how Satan attacked me when I was weak,
magnified the situation in my mind, and brought fear and
sadness. But too exhausted to recognize the enemy's trick, I
bought into it.

God, however, had a better plan. A card I received in the mail
that morning reminded me that Jesus, our Great Physician,
always has time for us and knows exactly how to mend us.
He knows the physical problems and the emotional turmoil
that torment us. He is a God of precision and wisdom and
will provide exactly what we need.

Hope from above settled into my soul, and I felt the love of Jesus encircle me like a giant bear hug. It was almost like He was personally whispering in my ear, "Be still and know that I am God."

God knows when we are too exhausted to fight. When we're too distraught to even reach out for His help, He is there. When we can no longer hold on, He cradles us securely in His loving arms.

In 1 Kings 19, the prophet Elijah—a mighty man of God—fearfully ran for his life. He fled to the desert, sat down under a tree, and prayed that he might die: "I've had enough, Lord. Take my life."

Elijah fell asleep and woke when an angel touched him and told him to get up and eat. There, beside him, was hot bread and water, prepared by the angel. Elijah ate and fell asleep again. A second time, the angel woke him and beckoned him to eat again, for "the journey is too much for you."

Again, he ate and drank. "Strengthened by that food, he traveled forty days and forty nights until he reached Horeb, the mountain of God."

At some point, we've probably echoed Elijah's thoughts. Maybe we haven't actually demanded that God take our lives, but instead, said something like, "I've had enough. I can't take any more."

Overwhelmed with the problems of life, we see no end and lose all desire to continue. But as He did for Elijah, God will meet our immediate needs of nourishment and rest until we are strengthened enough to continue.

We, too, can trust God to meet our needs, but according to His plan. Like manna in the wilderness, God promises enough grace for one day at a time. Enough comfort. Enough love.

And as we learn to keep our eyes on God's provision for today, fear of the future fades and hope takes its place.

"For our light and momentary troubles are achieving for us an eternal glory that far outweighs them all. So we fix our eyes not on what is seen, but on what is unseen. For what is seen is temporary, but what is unseen is eternal."

2 Corinthians 4:17-18

Writing from the Heart
Healing...from the Inside Out

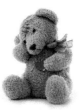

If feeling full of hope is a 5 and feeling totally hopeless is a 1, where do you fall on the scale right now? Write a letter to God explaining your answer.

It's one thing to say we believe that God has our best interest in mind, but how does your *heart* feel about this?

Why do you think David, in the book of Psalm, reminded himself so often of God's goodness and promise of deliverance?

And It Came to Pass

"Just because it doesn't make sense to you doesn't
mean it doesn't make sense."

Adrian Rogers

Finally, I thought. *I'm on the road to recovery.*

But this particular road still held many bumps to cross.
During my first evening home, I felt tight pressure in my
bowel. The pain increased as I tried, unsuccessfully, to relieve
myself.

"Lord, how could You be with me through so much and
leave me now? Okay. I know You didn't leave me, but how
can You let me suffer like this?"

By midnight, the pain was so intense I vomited repeatedly
and was taken back to the hospital. The emergency room
physician ordered tests, but I refused them. Just days out of
surgery, I couldn't tolerate the physical movement testing
would require.

I eventually convinced the charge nurse to telephone my OB-
GYN doctor and discovered he had just arrived at the
hospital for an emergency delivery. He would see me himself.

After an exam, he told me I was actually healing extremely
well—far beyond what he would have expected. My bowels

were working excellently. I just needed to wait for the process to take its course.

Still, I begged him not to send me home without relief. He took time to explain. "The bowel is putting pressure on all the other areas on which I operated. You need to take your meds consistently to stay ahead of the pain."

I did as I was told, and the process completed itself the next morning.

What God showed me was tremendous.

Though I questioned, or actually accused God of not caring, He was there all the time. He *had* never and *would* never back away because of any action on my part.

His presence was so very real and His part in meeting my needs so clear.

Despite the pain, I *was* healing. God never stopped working. He hadn't moved. I had simply allowed circumstances to block my view of Him.

God allows the stuff of life to rain on the righteous and the unrighteous. In fact, sometimes we wonder if it will ever pass. But we can rest assured; God is always in control.

He will not forsake us. He knows what we are going through, and He cares. We are precious in His sight. We may stumble at times, but He will always be there to pick us up and help us stand again.

Though we can't see it at the time, God is doing something in our lives. Trimming, shaping, firing—none of it enjoyable. Only God can determine how many cuts, how uncomfortable the situation, and how much debris needs to be removed.

Because only God can determine exactly how much work it will take to produce the results He desires.

Many times, when we don't understand what is happening to us physically, God reminds us of His love. And with that knowledge comes peace and the power to continue. Power to trust—at least until the next set back. But when and if that comes, Jesus will assure us of His love again. And again. Forever.

> "Being confident of this, that He who began a good work in you will carry it on to completion until the day of Christ Jesus."
>
> Philippians 1:6

Writing from the Heart
Healing...from the Inside Out

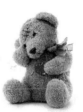

Maybe you know God would never overlook your need, but circumstances sure look otherwise. How does this make you feel?

Someone once said that *God loves us as we are but loves us too much to leave us that way.* In what ways can you see your trial as an act of God's love?

What do you need from God today? Be specific.

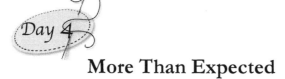

More Than Expected

"God loves each one of us as if there were only one of us."

Saint Augustine

Recovery was going to take a long time. Day after day, I struggled—lonely and discouraged. "Lord," I wrote. "I'm having a difficult time reaching Your presence."

Imagine my surprise when a response popped into my mind. Was God speaking to me?

My child, what do you think it means to cast your cares on Me?

"I thought it meant to trust You to take care of my situation. But, I think I was trying to do it my way ... just so I could believe that I believed. Now I wonder if it isn't more about taking time to tell You my fears, pain, and anxiety, without feeling guilty for needing Your love."

Why do you feel guilty for needing My love?

"Because I worry more about meeting my needs than those of others. I treasure my personal relationship with You and think of You mainly as a God who loves, comforts, and restores. But, sometimes, I wonder if I shouldn't stand back, blend into the crowd, and stop requiring Your individual attention. You deserve to be thought of as the King of kings. So why don't I feel that way?"

I created a void in you that desires My presence. I am what you desire to meet your needs. Love is not just one of My characteristics; I am love! Do you exalt or glorify anyone on earth?

"One of my previous pastors—such a man of God and full of love."

Did you admire and respect him before you knew his love?

"No. I've always known gentleness and goodness from him."

Did you have to force yourself to shift gears from knowing his love to admiring him?

"No. I don't feel awe toward him or anything, just a deep, loving appreciation for who he is and a respect for his wisdom and godly character. Sometimes I ache for the kind of love I hear in his voice but feel hopeless because I see no way of ever receiving that kind of love in my life. I'm not worth it. I'm nothing special."

Could I supply that love?

"Yes."

Do you think I want to do that?

"I want to believe that. I'm about to break down right now."

As we dialogue honestly with God, His persistent love breaks through like raindrops on parched ground, loosening resistant soil. But sadly, clumps of uncertainty form almost immediately. We want to believe in the depths of God's love, but some of us have never known stable, unconditional love, and we struggle to relate.

Gradually, as we come to understand that our feelings are based on faulty foundations, our hearts dare to open enough to receive God's love. To realize He doesn't parcel it out one dose at a time.

Rather, He showers us with the fullness of His love. For it is in His perfect and complete love that our needs are met. And as we cuddle in His embrace, we will naturally develop admiration and respect for His glorious majesty.

"See what great love the Father has lavished on us, that we should be called children of God! And that is what we are!"

1 John 3:1-3

Writing from the Heart
Healing...from the Inside Out

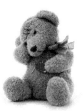

What beliefs do you have that could prevent you from totally opening yourself up to the fullness of God's love? Dig deeply.

Why is it critical for you to understand and remember that God's love is *unconditional?*

Write about a time when you were disappointed or wounded by someone in whose love you trusted. How might this affect your understanding of God's love?

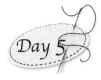

Take Two

> "If we have not quiet in our minds, outward comfort will do no more for us than a glass slipper on a gouty foot."
>
> John Bunyan

Three months after surgery, I still dealt with prolonged infection. Tests confirmed doctors' suspicions. Another surgery was necessary. I knew God would be with me, but I dreaded the intense pain.

On Saturday night, I went for a prayer walk and asked the Lord to send someone I could talk to. Someone who knew Him intimately. Someone I could trust to give scripturally based answers.

Sunday evening, as I played the piano after the service, a woman I didn't know approached, stood for a few minutes, then turned and left.

When I finished, friends invited me to go out for a sandwich, but I declined. My heart was heavy. I was so anxious about the upcoming surgery.

As I drove home, though, I felt impressed to go back. I knew the Lord was telling me to stop running from people, that I needed fellowship. Although everything in me said no, I obeyed.

At the restaurant, I took the last seat, next to the woman who had approached the piano. I'd never met her personally. She traveled as a Christian speaker and only visited our church occasionally.

She turned to face me. "How are you, Barb?"

"I'm fine, thanks."

"Are you nervous about your upcoming surgery?"

I guess she knows because Pastor asked for prayer. Still, she seems so loving and concerned—not like someone who doesn't even know me.

"Barb," she whispered. "Do you need someone to talk to?"

I nodded, unable to speak.

"During the service," she explained, "the Lord gave me a burden for you that was so heavy I couldn't stop weeping. I knew, immediately, that you needed someone to talk to. You were busy playing the piano after the service, and I thought I had missed the Lord's direction. But as I started to leave, the Holy Spirit touched my heart once again, and I knelt in the back to intercede for you a while longer."

We chatted a few minutes and arranged to meet again. God blessed my new friend with wisdom and insight as she listened and responded to my questions.

God's love is complete in every way. He understands our need to understand. Our desire to take the few pieces of the puzzle that we have and figure out the whole picture. Our innate desire/need to control the details of our lives.

But His perfect love has a better plan. One in which He carries the weight of such knowledge and control. One in which we cast our heavy burdens on Him, and He gives us rest.

Affliction has a way of bringing us to a point where we are so desperate for relief that we finally let go and let God take over. Where we come to the end of ourselves, admit our own inadequacies, and turn completely to God. And when we totally surrender and allow God to be God in our lives, our trust in Him grows, and His infinite love revives, refreshes, and restores our peace and joy.

"Your Father knows what you need before you ask Him."

Matthew 6:8

Writing from the Heart
Healing...from the Inside Out

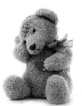

Sometimes we surrender a need to the Lord, only to take it right back. How can we keep this from happening so often?

If I hadn't obeyed God's nudge to return to the restaurant, I might have missed His provision. Why did God say, "To obey is better than sacrifice" in 1 Samuel 15:22?

In Revelation 1:10, the author writes, "On the Lord's Day I was in the Spirit, and I heard behind me a loud voice like a trumpet." John was positioned where he needed to be to hear from God. Similarly, the woman I mentioned above heard from God because she was in His presence. What keeps you from spending more time waiting in the presence of God to hear His still, small voice?

Week 4:

Invisible Stitch of Faith

"Faith is like radar that sees through the fog—the reality of things at a distance that the human eye cannot see."

Corrie Ten Boom

Just before my second surgery, I attended our church's family camp. During the first service, the leader introduced a minister's wife suffering from a severed Achilles tendon.

She sat in a wheelchair in short shorts, unable to tolerate clothing on her legs. Every service, ushers brought her forward for prayer. Three days into the week, she was miraculously healed and ran across the platform praising God. What a time of rejoicing!

I stood with the others in the auditorium, but on the inside I crumbled and hit bottom so hard I wondered if I would ever get up again.

Turmoil burned away at my soul. Scum. That's how I felt. How could I not be happy for this woman?

Oh, maybe I was happy for her; I just couldn't bear to think about her. I was eaten up with feelings of jealousy and rejection. You see, while conversation about God's goodness buzzed around me, I was still in great physical pain. I still had to face another surgery. *I* had prayed, and nothing had changed.

Those of us who cope with persistent pain often silently shudder when others give God glory for answers to prayer. Big answers. Small answers. We're tempted to give up.

We assume we don't have enough faith—or no faith at all. But in simply bringing our disbelief to God, we are signifying that we do. Faith that God can help us overcome our disbelief. Faith that answers to our questions can be found in Him.

Why does God delay in answering our prayers at times? Perhaps He is cleaning debris from our thought patterns to make room for our growing faith. Teaching us to focus on His character rather than what He can do for us. Training us to trust in His perfect timing as we wait. And shoring up our true identities—who we really are in Him.

In this week's lessons, we'll look closely at the subject of faith. We'll talk about how we are affected when God remains silent. We'll discuss the possibility of having faith like the woman with the issue of blood who touched Jesus' garment and was instantly healed.

We'll examine times we think our faith is gone, and discover that it's really not. Times when we are vulnerable to Satan's attacks on our emotions. And how we can resist the enemy as we focus on God's faithful love and protection.

Our faith will grow as we share an experience where God went above and beyond to reach out to a lonely, hurting child.

And as we develop a deeper understanding of true faith, we will be able to say along with James H. Aughey, "Christ is the Good Physician. There is no disease He cannot heal; no sin He cannot remove; no trouble He cannot help."

Yes, No, or Maybe . . . I Still Believe

"The issue of faith is not so much whether we believe in God, but whether we believe the God we believe in."

R.C. Sproul

When I was ten, the State Police called to say my older sister had been involved in an automobile accident. My dad sent me to the car to get his atlas. I prayed earnestly that my sister wouldn't die. I reminded God of the verse I'd recently memorized—Matthew 7:7. "Ask and it will be given to you; seek and you will find; knock and the door will be opened to you."

I knew God would answer my prayer. But then I heard my mother scream and saw her faint as I re-entered the house. My siblings said Gail had died.

I didn't believe them. God had promised: "Ask and it shall be given unto you."

But in reality, she was gone. Some said my sister received her *ultimate* healing. Just words to me. An adult's *acceptable* explanation for God's broken promise.

Fast-forward thirty years. I was recovering from a second surgery. Once again, God hadn't answered my prayers for healing. At least not in the way I expected. I wrote:

Lord, I know in my heart that I don't believe anymore. And I don't know how to start. I know you can heal me, but I guess I don't believe that you ever will. My faith is gone.

I felt guilty for not being able to believe. Not being able to muster up enough faith to *claim my healing*. Not being able to discern what sin I harbored in my heart that separated me from God's presence and rendered me ineligible to receive His healing.

Why include this story in the book? Because, as adults, it's critical that we realize our beliefs have been shaped by influences from the past—education, experience, parents, religious training, etc. Through the years we've patched opinions together to form our current stand. But the truth is, we need to carefully examine our beliefs in light of Scripture because many of them have faulty foundations. We need to be prepared to change our minds.

Can our lack of faith affect God's faithfulness to His promises? Romans 3:3-4a says, "What if some were unfaithful? Will their unfaithfulness nullify God's faithfulness? Not at all!"

Somewhere, in my past, I accepted a teaching that God *always* heals if we have enough faith. But as I examine that belief today, I must reject it. For you see, I have never, in my entire life, had as much faith in God's promise as I did the day my sister died.

And yet, God said no. Not because I didn't have enough faith. But because, in His divine sovereignty, He deemed it right.

Today, I readily pray for healing, in faith, believing that God, in His infinite wisdom and unfathomable love, will answer. I ask . . . and I keep on asking . . . until healing is received or death intervenes. For God does sometimes say no. But either way, my faith is secure because it rests not in the answer to my prayer but in my precious Lord and Savior.

"He Himself bore our sins in His body on the cross, so that we might die to sins and live for righteousness; by His wounds you have been healed."

1 Peter 2:24

Writing from the Heart

Healing...from the Inside Out

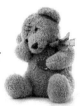

Describe a time when God failed to provide something very important for you or someone you know? How important is it to acknowledge and deal with the feeling of rejection?

Create a situation in which it would be wise for an adult to delay a response to a child's need or request. How could this reasoning apply to God's response to your prayers?

So often, when we're walking in pain, our beliefs about healing fluctuate and become muddled. One person tells us this. Another that. List everything you've ever heard about praying and believing for healing. Look up Scriptures to support or negate each point. Then take a stand. Ask God to guide you as you write a paragraph about what you believe the Bible says about healing.

Has Anyone Seen the Lord Lately?

"An infinite God can give all of Himself to each of His children. He does not distribute Himself that each may have a part, but to each one He gives all of Himself as fully as if there were no others."

A.W. Tozer

Faith seems to come in surges, then mysteriously shrinks away like the ocean tide. When we sense God's nearness and see prayers answered, our faith bank is refilled.

But what about when trials linger and we no longer feel the stir of the Holy Spirit as we worship? When we can't hear God's voice or feel His presence? Feeling abandoned at such a time, I wrote:

Lord, Your Word says that if I seek You, You will be found. I don't know any other way to seek You than to cry out to You. But it's not working.

Some time later, I attended a worship service where people all around were worshipping. Some weeping, others sweetly praising God's name in song and prayer.

I thought, "Lord, why am I not feeling anything? I know You're here and I'm not supposed to base everything on feelings, but others are obviously feeling You, and I want that, too."

I knew the Bible teaches that the Lord inhabits the praises of His people. "Okay, Lord," I prayed. "Feelings or not, I'm going to praise You."

As I shut my eyes and began giving thanks, I suddenly envisioned Jesus sitting with a crowd, ministering to them. I stood, as a small child, watching from a distance. I wanted so badly to be with Jesus. But, I thought, "No, He's busy, and they need Him right now. I need to stand back—it's not my time."

So I stayed put, yearning to touch Jesus.

Suddenly, Jesus looked my way. The love in His eyes was the only touch I needed. He had so much love for me. I started to cry, but Jesus didn't stop there. He got up from the crowd and walked over, picked me up, and carried me back to where He was sitting. I sat next to Him, and He put His arm around me and pulled me close.

I didn't want to leave. I could hardly believe Jesus was touching me. But after a few minutes, I sat up. "Lord, I need to go."

"Why?"

"Because all these people need your touch."

"Barbie," He said. "Do you know what omnipresent means?"

"Yes. Everywhere at the same time."

Jesus smiled. "You know what? I can be all things to all these people while I'm sitting here holding you. If you need to lie on My shoulder forever, it's okay. Don't leave."

So I sat in His presence, soaking up His love. His touch. His time.

Earlier God was silent. Why does He do this at times?

Perhaps He has something to say and is waiting for us to listen.

Perhaps we come to Him mainly with requests. So He steps back until we become hungry enough to seek His fellowship.

For God longs for us to run to His side, hug His neck, curl up in His embrace, and simply bask in His love. An intimate time where no words are needed. A time of silent comfort and joy and peace.

"He tends His flock like a shepherd: He gathers the lambs in His arms and carries them close to His heart."

Isaiah 40:11

Writing from the Heart
Healing...from the Inside Out

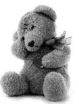

There are times when we don't feel like worshipping, but we do it anyway. Who do you think benefits more, God or us? Why?

If you could sit next to Jesus for an unlimited time, would you want to just rest in His embrace or to share your intimate secrets, questions, and needs? Explain your answer.

Describe the child who lives within you. Then rewrite Psalm 139:1-18 as a letter from God to your inner child.

Have You Heard the Good News?

"The greatest Christians in history seem to say that their sufferings ended up bringing them the closest to God—so this is the best thing that could happen, not the worst."

Peter Kreeft

At times I felt like the woman mentioned in Mark 5. "She had suffered a great deal under the care of many doctors and had spent all she had, yet instead of getting better she grew worse."

Not quite the abundant life God promises. In fact, I'll admit to a touch of anger. Okay, at least a dumpster full. Why was I so unworthy that God wouldn't choose to bless *me* just once? I'd done everything I knew to please Him. I wrote:

It's been so long, and I've asked so many times. I see other people prayed for and healed. That hurts, Lord. It's easier to not ask than to ask, get my hopes up, and then be disappointed yet another time. It feels like rejection, and frankly, I'd rather suffer the physical pain than risk the rejection of not being healed again.

Hoping to find answers, I continued reading. "When she heard about Jesus, she came up behind Him in the crowd and touched His cloak, because she thought, 'If I just touch His clothes, I will be healed.' Immediately her bleeding stopped and she felt in her body that she was freed from her suffering."

I'd like to say the passage strengthened my faith, but it didn't. I, too, had sincerely reached out to God with all my heart, but I still hurt. And I'd fallen prey to the myth that unanswered prayer equals personal rejection from God.

Instead of looking for Jesus, I was merely seeking to increase my faith enough to move the hand of God. Something *I* could do.

But, as Andrew Wommack explains, "The Lord doesn't look at [our] praying, confessing, begging, fasting, agreeing with others, and the other things [we] do as adding up to 'enough' to make Him move." Christ, alone, bore the stripes on His back at Calvary for our healing. We cannot, and must not, try to add to that.

The woman with the issue was sick for 12 years. Cast from society. Hopeless. Depressed. Yet, *when she heard about Jesus . . .* she summoned what little strength remained and set out to find Him.

The curious gathered around. The intrigued followed. The interested pressed in to hear more. But the desperate woman continued until she connected. And Jesus responded.

"Touching God requires that we draw close to Him and strive to enter into the realm of the spirit," says James May. "Just one touch of the Master's Hand will make all the difference in any situation."

Where did the woman get her faith? She *heard about Jesus.* Others were talking about this Jesus who healed diseases and cast out evil spirits. This Jesus who astonished the Synagogue leaders with His wisdom and insight. This Jesus who willingly walked among the lowly. This same Jesus who lives in our hearts and lives today.

Faith comes by hearing. Exploring God's Word and getting to know Jesus better every day. Drawing close enough to reach out and receive His healing touch.

> "Surely the arm of the Lord is not too short
> to save, nor His ear too dull to hear."
>
> Isaiah 59:1

Writing from the Heart
Healing...from the Inside Out

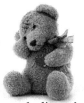

Do you think faith and doubt can co-exist in a believer's heart? If they can, should they? Why or why not? How could this "all-or-nothing" mindset be dangerous to your perception of God's grace?

Have you ever felt like God would answer more of your prayers if you were a better Christian? What would this look like in real life? How do you think God would respond to your answer?

Where would you rate your prayer life—with the curious who gathered, the intrigued who followed, the interested who pressed in to hear more, or the desperate woman who continue until she connected? In what way might your placement fluctuate as life's circumstances change?

Time for a Lube Job

"Faith is deliberate confidence in the character of God whose ways you may not understand at the time."

Oswald Chambers

The time came to have my second surgery. God had provided all that I needed to prepare myself emotionally. I wasn't worried. I really was going to be okay.

A few nights before, I attended a wiener roast with my church family. As several friends gathered around, we began to talk about "lady things." Well, this got funnier as we went. At some point, we came up with the idea of finding one of those little vinyl stickers they put on your windshield when you have your oil changed, and putting it on my abdomen when I was ready to go to surgery.

I didn't get around to picking one of those up, so I improvised and made a set of musical notes from an index card—appropriate because my doctor was an avid piano player. On the bar across the top of the notes, I wrote "A couple of notes for the doctor." On one of the notes, I wrote, "Go easy on the tape," and on the other, "Please don't stretch anything you just tightened in the last surgery."

Then, at the very bottom, I added a request based on a certain dryness I had experienced since the previously performed hysterectomy. In small letters, I wrote, "While you're at it, could you please give me a lube job?"

I attached the notes to my belly and let the surgical nurse in on the prank before I fell asleep. When I woke up in recovery, the nurse read my bandage to me: "Lube Job Included!" Who says surgery can't be fun?

Well, maybe that part of the surgery was fun. But what about those first few days after surgery when infection set in and I still couldn't void completely? I'll be honest. My faith took a major nosedive. I felt so angry that God let me down again. How could I even face Him with the ugliness in my soul?

Satan knows our vulnerability and takes advantage of it in times of weakness. Convinces us to stop seeking. Stop praying. Stop hoping.

Guilt. Shame. Lies. God loves another person more than you. You are not worthy of God's touch. You have sin in your life. Your prayers make no difference to God.

Hebrews 10:22 says, "Let us draw near to God with a sincere heart and with the full assurance that faith brings, having our hearts sprinkled to cleanse us from a guilty conscience and having our bodies washed with pure water."

It's in these times we must turn to God with total honesty. Confess our doubt and shame. Draw near to Him with sincere hearts. Just like the verse instructs.

We don't want to hide from God. That would play right into Satan's hand. The Lord knows our every thought, anyway. He understands completely. As we confess our lack of trust, He will walk us through our confusion and sprinkle our hearts to cleanse us. He will encourage us, restore our faith, and in time, make us whole.

"Search me, O God, and know my heart; test me and know
my anxious thoughts. See if there is any offensive
way in me, and lead me in the way everlasting."

Psalm 139:23-24

Writing from the Heart

Healing...from the Inside Out

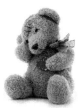

Being one of the last to be chosen for something is a painful
experience, not soon forgotten. Have you ever been jealous
when someone else's prayer gets answered and you're still
waiting to hear from God on yours? Describe how that feels.

Why do you think God answers some prayers quickly and
doesn't seem to respond at all to others? Can you do anything
to change that?

God promises to bless us abundantly. How might the
blessings He's referring to differ from what we usually picture
in our minds?

I Don't Believe in Suicide, But . . .

"One of the things I have learned from severe pain is that I have felt totally abandoned by God . . . Maybe that's what makes it so sweet after the pain goes and the Lord says, 'I was here all the time. I haven't left you. I will never forsake you.'"

Joyce Landorf

The second surgery failed.

As I begged God to show me what I was doing wrong, I pictured Him standing over me, waiting for me to get my act together so He could heal me.

Confusion led to depression. I kept thinking how wonderful death must be. I told friends not to feel sorry if I died because life wasn't worth living anyway. Surely in heaven I could do things right, and God would be pleased with me.

I knew suicide was wrong, and I never contemplated it. But I did decide not to seek further medical help. Maybe my physical problems would get so bad they would actually take my life.

This was the only path to take. I couldn't handle the emotional pain and rejection if God, once again, chose not to provide my healing.

At this time, a dear friend wrote me a letter—the Holy Spirit guiding her hand.

My precious friend, as I've been reasoning with the Father about you and the situation you are in, many things have come to mind. I thought about my own children and would I want to see them endure almost unbearable pain; and did not Jesus bear our pain in His own body on the cross; and if He bore our pain, would He desire for us to bear it as well? One who loves us so much, would He desire that we suffer?

My thoughts went to Job and I realized the great fight of affliction that God entrusted him with. God knew something about this man, and God said to Satan, "Have you considered my servant Job?" Satan said, "You've got a hedge about him and I can't get to him." God said, "See, he's in your hands." God knew what was in Job and my sweet and precious sister, He knows you. Could it be that He has entrusted you with a great fight of affliction because He knows what is in you?

I don't know the answers or the reasons, for He has not revealed them to me, but He knows. He knows you. You'll come through as gold tried in the furnace. He will bless your latter end more than your first.

I literally felt God's love in these words. I wept openly as I poured out my deepest feelings and felt God's tender loving kindness wash over me.

As we focus on God's love and protection, fear and despair begin to subside, replaced with faith and confidence that God will see us through.

In the midst of our trials, God will make Himself known in undeniable ways. He will use our struggles to lead us straight into His waiting arms. For it is there we learn to trust in His love and faithfulness. It is there we are reminded that He is our strength, our power, and our peace.

And it is there that in some small way, our trials begin to make just a little bit of sense.

"No temptation has overtaken you except what is common to mankind. And God is faithful; He will not let you be tempted beyond what you can bear. But when you are tempted, He will also provide a way out so that you can endure it."

1 Corinthians 10:13

Writing from the Heart

Healing...from the Inside Out

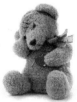

Do you ever find yourself emotionally numb when you pray—unable to connect with your pain? Why do you think this happens?

Describe a time when you decided to give up. What sent you over the edge? Did you sense the crisis coming? Could you have done anything to change the situation?

Read Job 1. Do you believe God automatically builds a hedge around each of His children as Satan claimed God had done for Job? Find scriptural support for your answer.

Week 5:

A Blind Stitch in the Dark

"Darkness cannot drive out darkness; only light can do that."
Martin Luther King, Jr.

I once attended a weekend conference where the speaker taught about living on eagle's wings—enjoying the privileges and promises we have as God's children. The following Monday morning I couldn't find my car keys. My frustration grew as I ran back and forth to the car trying spare keys I found around the house.

"C-a-w! C-a-w!" I looked up to find a huge black crow in my yard staring curiously at me. Instantly, I remembered the speaker asking the audience if we were going to continue living like crows, pecking for worms, or rise above the storm and soar like eagles. Laughter bubbled up within me, and my spirit lifted. The problem was still there, but the immensity of it faded immediately.

Bob Newhart once said, "Laughter gives us distance. It allows us to step back from an event, deal with it and then move on."

Focus. Perspective. Both critical when we are living with daily pain. Too often, tunnel vision takes over, and we can't see the forest for the trees. Life becomes simply the next step we take. This narrow point of view, along with unrealistic expectations, leaves little room for optimism and hope.

This week's lessons include an example of how a dirty lens can distort our view and affect our logic. How, many times, we don't even realize the glass is dirty . . . until we face a bright light and our vision is completely obstructed. We'll relate this to our understanding of what is happening in our lives. What God *is* or *is not* doing in response to our prayers. What we have to look forward to in the future.

We'll discuss the discomfort of walking in the dark—never sure where we are going, afraid of being caught off guard. And we'll note how the inability to control our pain often precipitates a need to micro-manage the rest of our world.

God promises peace if we keep our minds on Him. We'll talk about how to do that when pain and discouragement bombard our minds, and we'll see how God's creative love showed up in a tense, seemingly impossible situation.

We'll touch on the subject of depression. Huge topic, I know. But bottom line, we know that God understands and doesn't condemn us for our hopelessness. God created us and recognizes the frail state of our dust-formed bodies and minds. We'll study David's depressed thoughts in the book of Psalms and how he worked hard not to allow the feelings to dominate his life.

Finally, we'll explore the ultimate darkness of the enemy and how it threatens to take over our lives. To convince us to give up and end it all. But we won't stop there. There is a light brighter than any darkness Satan can ever generate. Jesus— the True Light.

With the Lord in our lives, we can say with the psalmist David, "The Lord is my light and my salvation—whom shall I fear? The Lord is the stronghold of my life—of whom shall I be afraid?" (Psalm 27:1)

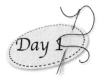

Double Vision

"There are two kinds of light—the glow that illuminates,
and the glare that obscures."

James Thurber

There are many times when we think we see the whole picture clearly. But, in reality, we see only from a cloudy point of view. I Corinthians 13:12 explains, "Now we see but a poor reflection as in a mirror; then we shall see face to face. Now I know in part; then I shall know fully, even as I am fully known."

This verse came to life one morning on my way to work. As I turned my car toward the sun, I was suddenly unable to see through a windshield that had seemed clean just a few seconds before. Glaring rays of sunlight ricocheted off dirt and grime, impeding my vision until I turned the corner and could see clearly once again.

My direction was the only thing that changed. The dirt was still present. I just couldn't see it when I turned away from the light.

God taught me so much through that experience. I thought I understood where He was going. I thought I had things figured out. Then, when another surgery became necessary, it threw me for a loop. How could God allow this when I was just starting to heal from the previous surgery?

The Lord asked me to simply trust Him. He pointed out that if I began to rely on my own understanding, I would be placing myself in jeopardy. There was dirt on my glass that I could not see. He promised that when I turned my eyes upon Jesus, His light would reveal darkness in my life that needed to be cleaned.

Gradually, I began to understand why 2 Corinthians 5:7 instructs us to "live by faith, not by sight."

God sees the whole picture. Clearly—without obstructions.

We know that. But sometimes, in the midst of our problems, the dirt on our glass—pain, doubt, and discouragement— impairs our vision, distorting the picture and muddling reality.

Think of a dark hotel room. We flip on the bathroom light in the night, and it blinds us. Our eyes have become accustomed to the dark.

That's the way it is with God's light. He lovingly controls the intensity because He understands where we are and how much light we can tolerate at one time. However, as we continue to focus on Him, our eyes will adjust and our vision will become clear and true.

What are *we* to do? Surrender the internal drive to control our own lives. Strive not to lean on our own limited vision and understanding. And trust completely in God, who promises in Isaiah 42:16 to guide us along paths, turn darkness into light before us, and make our rough places smooth.

As we trust this promise, we find new hope—a flicker of light at the end of our dark, frightening tunnel that will guide us all the way.

"When Jesus spoke again to the people, He said, 'I am the light of the world. Whoever follows me will never walk in darkness, but will have the light of life.'"

John 8:12

Writing from the Heart

Healing...from the Inside Out

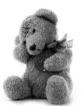

How is living with chronic pain similar to walking in the dark?

What is it that makes walking in the dark so scary? How could the fear of stumbling or being caught off guard affect your walk with the Lord?

When we face the light of God, we can see the dirt in our lives—faulty perceptions, a narrow point of view, etc. What does God want us to do about these?

A Starr Experience

"Our prayers lay the track down which God's power can come. Like a mighty locomotive, His power is irresistible, but it cannot reach us without the rails."

Watchman Nee

I was one of those kids who actually enjoyed piano lessons. So when brilliant classical piano music met me at the door of the doctor's office, I smiled and said, "I hope you're good, Doc, because I like you already."

The doctor eagerly described the grand piano he had recently purchased. "My friends and I are giving a recital," he said. "You're welcome to attend if you feel up to it."

I hadn't played seriously for years, but attending the recital just weeks after my first surgery rekindled my passion. I went home and played for hours.

Unfortunately, my piano couldn't compete with my speed. I often returned to keys not yet ready to replay. As soon as I was able, I went shopping and fell in love with a Yamaha concert grand. My husband gasped at the price. "Sure," he said. "You can buy a new one—as soon as you sell the one we have."

The year before, he'd bought a dilapidated baby grand from a swap shop, refinished the body, and paid to have the action, strings, and keys redone. Result? A gorgeous piano with an *average* action.

Needless to say, we had a few dollars invested. "Father," I prayed. "Buying this piano would be a huge investment. Our money is Your money, so please let us know Your will. If our piano doesn't sell in seven days, I'm going to believe You want us to keep it. On the other hand, if it sells, I'm trusting that You are giving Your okay to buy the new one."

As soon as I finished, the music store called. "You mentioned you have a Starr piano. The name sounded familiar, so I checked my records. A woman has been calling for almost two years looking for a Starr grand piano. The company belonged to her husband's grandfather."

I sold our piano that night and bought the Yamaha the next day. I'm still amazed at how God orchestrated this experience. What were the odds I would call that huge store and *happen* to speak to the same clerk Mrs. Starr had been contacting?

God knew the desire of my heart. I wanted to purchase a piano equal to my ability. But even more, I wanted to walk in God's will.

In Bible times, Jews expected the Messiah to be a mighty conqueror. Locked in to what they *expected*, many completely missed the humble appearance of Jesus.

We must be careful not to do the same when we pray. Requests and decisions become confusing and difficult when we don't feel well. But if we predetermine the exact answer we are looking for in our prayer, we risk misreading God's answer or missing it completely.

Instead, let's remember that God often answers in a manner or direction totally different than that which we expect. And, of course, His way far exceeds anything we could ever imagine or think!

> "And we know that in all things God works for the good of those who love Him, who have been called according to His purpose."
>
> Romans 8:28

Writing from the Heart
Healing...from the Inside Out

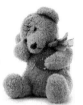

Though useless in my eyes, the STARR piano was the very desire of Mrs. Starr's heart. What does God's willingness to minister uniquely to individual desires say about His love?

Can you think of a time when God came through just in the knick of time for you or someone you know? Write about the experience and allow the memory to bolster your faith in God's perfect plan and timing.

Chronic pain often leads to a general sense of apathy for the things we used to love. Is there a hobby or activity you've lost interest in because of your pain? Returning to this love often rekindles a spark of renewed joy and excitement for life within you. Can you commit to spending at least twenty minutes a day to give this a try?

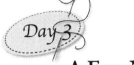

A Few Notes About Peace

"Faith sees the invisible, believes the unbelievable,
and receives the impossible."

Corrie Ten Boom

During the weeks after my second surgery, I spent hours practicing for the upcoming recital. I was ready, but incredibly nervous.

The night before the recital, my husband and I attended a church dinner and worship service. My mind, however, was on my performance. I longed to be home practicing.

But as the praise music began, I reconsidered and prayed, "This stress isn't worth it, Lord. I don't want to miss this time with You. I'll just skip the recital."

The next morning, I talked to God. "You know I want to perform today, and You promised to keep me in perfect peace when my mind is stayed on You. But how do I play classical music *and* keep my mind on You?"

I fingered the first few notes of a Chopin waltz, and the most amazing thing happened. As I ended the first line with ascending chords, I sensed the Lord singing, "I am your Lord" to the tune of the music. My spirit quickened. The music changed to a gentle swing, and I pictured myself as a child, waltzing through a flower garden with Jesus.

The next passage featured a strong rolling section with the left hand and ended with a long, difficult run up the piano with my right hand. As I began, I envisioned myself sitting in a small boat on a stormy sea, rocking back and forth violently. But just as the boat threatened to tip, Jesus stood. That was the run with my right hand. I'd never executed the run like I did that time. My fingers were flying!

I went to the recital, and the Holy Spirit again brought one heavenly encounter after another to mind as I played. Sweet communion with the Lord.

Philippians 4:6-7 says, "Do not be anxious about anything, but in everything, by prayer and petition, with thanksgiving, present your requests to God. And the peace of God, which transcends all understanding, will guard your hearts and your minds in Christ Jesus."

Do not be anxious. Like we have a choice? Like we can control feelings?

Of course not. God understands there will be times when peace eludes us. Like times when physical pain flares, and we see no end in sight. When we are exhausted and overcome with discouragement.

But He wants us to know there is a way out. We might compare the process to changing the oil in an automobile. Before servicemen add clean, fresh oil, they must allow time for the old oil to drain until the tank is completely empty.

God says that when we do feel anxious, He wants us to refocus. Come and talk to Him. Tell Him what we need. Thank Him for His provision, His promises, and His presence. And when we've completely emptied our anxiety onto His shoulders, He will refill the void with His peace.

When anxiety builds, remember the recital. Keep your mind on God, and He will creatively supply all that you need in ways you have yet to even imagine.

"The Lord your God is in your midst, a mighty one who will save; He will rejoice over you with gladness; He will quiet you by His love; He will exult over you with loud singing."

Zephaniah 3:17

Writing from the Heart
Healing...from the Inside Out

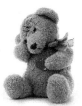

Anxiety has a way of rudely overtaking all other thoughts and feelings. Write a letter to God explaining what makes you anxious and why. Empty your tank. What are you afraid of? What do you dread? Ask God how you can keep your mind on Him when in a particularly anxious situation.

Waiting on test results can often produce anxiety. But can worry change anything? What activities could you participate in to redirect your thoughts once you've specifically surrendered your anxious feelings to God?

Unable to control our physical pain, we crave to get a handle on the rest of our world—to make sense of and create order in our everyday lives. Unfortunately, even if we do manage this, we have to figure out how to maintain the order. How has your situation affected your need for some sort of control in life?

Day 4

Feelings Object. Faith Answers

"God is more concerned with conforming me to the likeness of His Son than leaving me in my comfort zones."

Joni Eareckson Tada

Finally, two months after my second surgery, I was referred to the right doctor—a uro-gynecologist who alleviated much of my pain with injections and physical therapy. He explained that only a physician trained in urology *and* gynecology could adequately understand the complexity of my problems.

Then life threw another curve. My husband received military relocation orders. I did the research. No uro-gynecologists within a hundred miles of our new home.

I was afraid to admit how angry I was with God. I tried to remember the lessons I'd been learning, but nothing seemed to help. Once again, I wrote a letter to God.

Feelings. Emotions. I can't seem to control these. One day I'm up and the next day I'm on bottom. I feel guilty about not being stable. If my relationship is right with You, shouldn't I be experiencing peace and joy all the time?

Father, You said You are the same yesterday, today, and forever. Does that mean that with Your help, it is possible for me to remain steady every day?

You've spoken to me about thinking about positive things. When I dwell on how bad things are, I really go down fast. I'm trying to control this, Lord. But I don't know what to do when I wake up depressed. When I feel this heavy oppression or weight on my shoulders. How do I cast this burden on You? How do I do it? It's so heavy.

Now, on top of physical pain, I struggled with emotional pain. Guilt. Shame. How could I be depressed as a Christian?

The Lord came to my rescue by showing me 2 Corinthians 7:6 where it says, "God comforts the downcast." From the Greek word *tapeinos*, downcast means depressed, base, or lowly.

So, if God recognizes our bodies are imperfect and promises to love and comfort us through these experiences, it must not be a sin for a Christian to be downcast or depressed at times.

In Psalm 42, David asks three times, "Why so downcast, O my soul?" David first tries to self-correct his feelings, saying, "Why so downcast, O my soul? Put your hope in God, for I will yet praise Him, my Savior and my God."

When that didn't work, He turned to God for help. In verse six, he says, "My soul is downcast within me; therefore I will remember You from the land of the Jordan, the heights of Hermon—from Mount Mizar." David's hiding places. He reminded himself that God was with him wherever he went.

Matthew Henry, a great Bible commentator, notes that in this passage, feelings object and faith answers.

So often, we deplete our strength trying to ignore our feelings and continue as if life is fine—ashamed that we can't consistently walk in God's peace.

But we can learn from David's response as we acknowledge our feelings and redirect our thoughts. Verbally command our souls to focus on God's presence and power, and allow faith to trump our feelings.

"Praise the Lord, my soul, and forget not all His benefits— who forgives all your sins and heals all your diseases, who redeems your life from the pit and crowns you with love and compassion, who satisfies your desires with good things so that your youth is renewed like the eagle's."

Psalm 103:2-5

Writing from the Heart

Healing...from the Inside Out

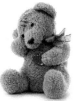

How did David find balance between acknowledging his feelings and dwelling on them in Psalm 42?

Each repetition of an echo fades slightly until the original sound is gone. How could sharing your emotional pain with others result in the same sort of fading-echo effect?

Prayer or Prozac? Does it really have to be one or the other? As Christians, many of us balk at taking medicine to help balance our emotions. But we have no problem wearing glasses or taking medicine for Diabetes. What is the difference? Is there really anything un-Christian about taking anti-depressants?

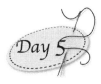

True Light

"In order for the light to shine so brightly,
the darkness must be present."

Francis Bacon

Pain is darkness. So is doubt, bitterness, hopelessness, and anger. But at times, these feelings become so familiar we actually welcome them as friends. We hesitate to embrace change, not sure we're ready to face the unknown.

Fortunately, the darkness doesn't surprise God. He urges us to bring our cares to Him because He desires to relieve the pent-up pain and lessen the potential risk of a hardened heart.

Darkness threatened to smother me one night when I headed to bed with a migraine. The pain medicine hadn't worked. *Swallow the whole bottle of pills. Then the pain will go away.*

I sensed an evil presence. "Lord, help me," I prayed. With a warm cloth on my forehead, I massaged my eyes. The pain was intense. "What can I do to stop it, Lord?"

"Lay down the cloth," He whispered to my spirit.

"I don't understand. That's the only thing that is helping."

"Trust me."

As I put the cloth down, turned over to rest, and shut my eyes, my pillow instantly felt firm and I felt myself nestled in the Lord's embrace. As I cried on His strong shoulder, I kept hearing "the blood of Jesus" in my mind, over and over again. Then I literally felt what I believe was Jesus gently rubbing oil over the aching bones around my eyes. The pain eased and within minutes, I fell asleep.

If I'd never known such darkness, I'd never have known Light to the degree I then did. The darkness led me to the Light of the world, and instantly, the Light—Jesus—dispelled the darkness around and within me. As the Lord gave the words, I penned the following.

> *True Light shines best in darkness.*
>
> *Isolation. Loneliness. Pain.*
>
> *For where other light is present, True Light is sadly misperceived.*
>
> *Unnecessary. Incomprehensible. Nonexistent.*
>
> *Other light, though truly begotten by True Light,*
>
> *Fades into deception as it creeps from its source, seeking a dim path of its own.*
>
> *Glory to pride. Knowledge to ignorance. Revelation to confusion.*
>
> *Darkness demands a real answer.*
>
> *A way out.*
>
> *A source with eternal power behind it.*
>
> *A Light that will outshine all others in the deepest chasm.*
>
> *True Light preceded, surpasses, and dispels darkness.*
>
> *Jesus said, "I am the Light of the world."*
>
> *Forever.*

No wonder God allows dark patches in our lives. For as we carefully navigate the obscure path before us, we instinctively focus on the Light, and God is able to reveal His love, His faithfulness, and His inexpressible glory.

"If I say, 'Surely the darkness will hide me and the light become night around me,' even the darkness will not be dark to You; the night will shine like the day, for darkness is as light to You."

Psalm 139:11-12

Writing from the Heart
Healing...from the Inside Out

Describe the darkest hour in your life. Did you see it coming? Where did you turn for help?

Has God ever asked you or someone you know to do something directly opposite from what you sincerely thought would be best? Did you follow through?

Most of the time, God provides just enough light for us to find our next few steps. How much do you worry about the path beyond that? Can worrying about the future actually cause more problems in your life today?

Week 6:

Overcast Seam of Feelings

"When you cannot rejoice in feelings, circumstances
or conditions, rejoice in the Lord."

A.B. Simpson

Feelings—frustration, anger, guilt, shame. As we walk
through our struggle for health, we battle these feelings
constantly.

One time I became angry with someone who wronged me
and allowed that anger to simmer for several days. I knew I
was handling the situation incorrectly, but felt somewhat
justified.

"Lord," I prayed, "that person just brings out the worst in
me."

"What's the worst doing in you?" the Lord asked.

Yikes! I didn't expect that response. But it's true, isn't it?
Many times, the Lord uses the trials in our lives to reveal the
worst within us so we will deal with it.

As pain continued to wrack my body, I became emotionally
and physically weak. I felt guilty because every time I hit my
knees to pray, I crumbled. The warm love of God's presence

instantly melted my shell, and with no walls to restrain it, sadness flowed uncontrollably.

The focus was on me. No worship or praise. No interceding for others. Just me and my problems. This went against everything I thought I knew about *Christ-like* prayer.

As I apologized to God for my pathetic prayer life, He totally surprised me by saying, "If you don't allow Me to cleanse the pain you kneel with, the love and power I pour into you for others will be weakened—tainted with self. You will be offering others a drink of cold water from a dirty cup."

I began to examine my feelings. An experience quickly popped into my mind. I'd asked for prayer, and a dear Christian friend said, "I will pray, but because you are a mature Christian, I feel I should point out that you are causing this pain yourself by trusting doctors instead of God for your healing and by taking medicine that harms your body."

Wow. Talk about condemnation. That one stuck. Though I strongly disagreed with her, a seed of doubt and shame had been planted.

The power of words. Hope and encouragement from friends. Life and promise from God. And, unfortunately, condemnation and death from Satan.

Then there's false guilt. That bad feeling that surfaces even when we've actually done nothing wrong. That ugly finger that attacks our very soul.

Satan jumps on our vulnerability and stands, as prosecutor, to deliver false claims about us. But instead of countering, we merely nod in agreement. In essence, accepting the claims without the slightest objection. And, thus, our self-inflicted punishment begins—joy and peace replaced by shame and condemnation.

Jesus once asked an invalid if he wanted to get well. In this week's lessons, we'll discuss the risk of succumbing to a victim mentality and what responsibility we play in avoiding this. Then we'll talk about surrendering our self-made strength for God's unlimited strength.

We'll explain how feelings follow thoughts. And we'll learn how to uncover and reject false beliefs by checking the validity of our thoughts under the scrutinizing light of Scripture.

Finally, we'll compare condemnation and conviction, how each affects us, and how to avoid negative feelings from budding and growing into bitterness. How to choose light over darkness. Life over death.

Nobody Knows the Trouble I've Seen

"Courage is being scared to death—but saddling up anyway."

John Wayne

Life can be so uncomfortable for those with chronic pain. Even the slightest activity triggers inflammation. Negative side effects often accompany prescription medications.

We hurt, day after day, and our thinking often becomes muddled. We might even take on victim mentalities. Nobody knows. Nobody cares. Darkness invades our souls as we lock ourselves away in that cold, lonely world of hopelessness.

But in 1 John 1:5, we are clearly instructed to rid ourselves of this darkness. "This is the message we have heard from Him and declare to you: God is light; in Him there is no darkness at all. If we claim to have fellowship with Him yet walk in the darkness, we lie and do not live by the truth. But if we walk in the light, as He is in the light, we have fellowship with one another, and the blood of Jesus, His Son, purifies us from all sin."

When Jesus approached an invalid beside the Pool of Bethesda and learned that the man had been in this condition for a long time, Jesus asked, "Do you want to get well?"

Sounds crazy, but is it really? The Word says that if we walk in darkness, we lie and do not live by the truth—the very truth that promises to set us free. Yet we continue to isolate ourselves, choosing to remain in the grips of death itself.

I want to be sensitive here. We're weak. We've been beaten down by pain for a long time. Sometimes survival is the most we can hope for. We've tried to fight in the battle, but we've fallen and don't believe we'll ever stand again.

Too often, says Helen Wodehouse, "we think we must climb to a certain height of goodness before we can reach God. But . . . if we are in a hole, the Way begins in the hole. The moment we set our face in the same direction as His, we are walking with God."

I'm not suggesting we make radical changes. Just that we look around, acknowledge where we are, and take the tiniest step toward the Light.

God, who yearns to minister to us in these times, calls gently. "Come to Me, all you who are weary and burdened, and I will give you rest" (Matthew 11:28). He covets our transparent honesty, for He knows the destructive power of unacknowledged doubt and despondency.

And greater still, He knows the healing power, mercy, and grace we receive when we choose to face our pain and confusion in the safety of His loving embrace.

He will keep His promises. But we, too, have responsibility. We come, and He will give us rest. We hope, and He will renew our strength.

God will shine His light as we take each step. And in His time—as perfect as with that of each day's magnificent sunrise—God, Himself, will dispel the darkness around us and replace it with the pure light of His love and grace.

"Let him who walks in the dark, who has no light,
trust in the name of the Lord and rely on his God."

Isaiah 50:10

Writing from the Heart

Healing…from the Inside Out

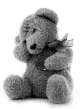

In what ways have you isolated yourself from others emotionally? Maybe you change the subject when others ask how you are doing or stay too busy to entertain relationships.

What feelings, thoughts, or circumstances cause you to shrink away in isolation? How could you use these to actually draw you closer to God? To others?

What practical steps can you take to focus more on God's grace than on your problems?

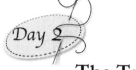

The Truth About Lies

"A lie is like a snowball; the further you
roll it the bigger it becomes."

Martin Luther

As I reestablished myself with Texas doctors, I wondered whether life was worth the effort. Succumbing to the overwhelming feelings of helplessness seemed so much easier than searching for faith and strength.

When I visited a doctor for ongoing migraines, she asked how I was doing emotionally. She was so kind and caring. I fell apart, and she suggested I see a mental health counselor for depression.

Once again, I asked myself how a Christian seeking God in prayer and spending time in the Bible could possibly be depressed. Hadn't I heard that faith and doubt could not co-exist? Further, if I entertained doubt in my heart, I surely had no faith. And without faith it was impossible to please God.

Totally confused, I gave in to my fears and located the correct office to schedule an appointment. There were no openings with military doctors, so the clerk asked my preference for an off-base doctor. I had no idea. I just knew that I would only agree to talk to a Christian therapist. As I contemplated my answer, the clerk replied, "Maybe I can recommend a solid Christian doctor."

According to strict military guidelines, she was not allowed to recommend one doctor over another. But she did.

God provided the wisest, most loving Christian doctor and therapist, whose counsel over the next few years changed everything in my life. I learned that my feelings follow my thoughts and beliefs. And I learned to recognize, identify, and reject false beliefs.

For example, if we believe that God is disappointed in us and has turned His face, we feel rejected when we don't see our prayers answered. But as we learn to base our thoughts and beliefs on the Word of God—that God does and always will care deeply for us—our feelings change. We begin to trust again.

At times, Satan initially snags us with the truth, and then twists it with a lie. He tells us we are not worthy of God's love. That's actually the truth. But he also convinces us that we have to do something or be something to earn God's love. That is a lie.

2 Corinthians 10:5 says, "We demolish arguments and every pretension that sets itself up against the knowledge of God, and we take captive every thought to make it obedient to Christ." Only as we carefully examine our thoughts on a daily basis to filter out the lies, will the truth be able to set us free.

While it may take a long time to change faulty thinking, it takes only a second to gaze into Jesus' eyes and know that we are being deceived. Only a second to realize those thoughts come from the pit of hell and that God loves us, even in our weakness. Especially in our weakness.

For when we are engulfed in darkness, He is our light. When we are drowning in sorrow, He is our comfort. And when we are too weak to stand, He is our strength.

If we allow God to purify our hearts, we will see Him, and He will heal us.

"Blessed are the pure in heart, for they will see God."

Matthew 5:8

Writing from the Heart

Healing...from the Inside Out

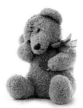

Why do you think we still have anxiety, even though we pray, read our Bibles, and attend church?

Feelings follow. As we change the way we think, our feelings will line up. Write about a situation in which you were disappointed, angry, or frustrated with someone. How did your thoughts influence your feelings?

Make a list of at least 10 reasons why life is and always will be worth the living.

Lord, Take My Spinach and Give Me Your Spirit

"Natural strength is what we receive from the hand of God as Creator. Spiritual strength is what we receive from God in grace."

Watchman-Nee

From an early age, we strive to be strong—independent and self-sufficient. To function without signs of stress. Weakness, we believe, implies an inadequacy or a need to be stronger.

One day I sat by a table in my first grade classroom. It was Parent Appreciation Day, and the students were showing their parents around the room. As I rested my arm on the back of a chair, one darling student shouted, "Hey, look at Mrs. Haley's muscle. No wonder she's so strong!"

Of course, what this child failed to realize was that most muscles are located on top of the arm, not hanging underneath. To say I was embarrassed wouldn't come close as the whole roomful of people turned to inspect the blob hanging below my arm.

In reality, I've always been strong. I have a high pain tolerance and can disguise my feelings well.

Throughout my physical battle, I tried to remain strong for the Lord. I tried to believe He was working behind the scenes. I tried to avoid dwelling on my problems as I concentrated on God's faithfulness. That seemed good.

From the beginning, I realized that sharing my pain with others caused me to focus more on my circumstances. And that quickly zapped my faith. Or what I believed was faith.

Actually, I think it was more about my ability to control my situation. My ability to appear strong by ignoring the weakness within. Some call it denial. I called it a logical choice. Survival.

You see, when our bodies suffer, we yearn for understanding and compassion. But in the end, a sympathetic ear is not really enough. After we share our woes and others express support and promise to pray, we walk away physically unchanged. We still hurt, and our minds are once again trained on the giants of the situation.

But life must go on, so we pack away the discouragement and hopelessness. The problem is, as our feelings become more difficult to bundle and manipulate, we begin to lose control. And we realize our strength is nothing but a sandy foundation that has deteriorated and left us weak and needy.

Perhaps…right where God wants us. Ready to hear the truth—that our ability to stay strong *for* the Lord is not at all what He desires.

Maybe God uses trials to reveal just how self-reliant we have become. To scrape off layers of pretense and skewed thinking behind what we call strength. To strip away pride and bring us to a point of true surrender to His life-changing power.

When God says, "Be strong," He's referring to something much more powerful than *self-produced* strength. In fact, He often allows circumstances in our lives that will deplete our strength so we will know the limits thereof and can be introduced to His *supernatural* strength that knows no limit.

"The Lord is my strength and my defense; He has become my salvation. He is my God, and I will praise Him, my father's God, and I will exalt Him."

Exodus 15:2

Writing from the Heart

Healing...from the Inside Out

Describe an experience in which you pretended to be strong but were hurting inside. Did you do this to protect yourself, others, or both? Explain.

When we try to be strong *for* the Lord, we are usually trying to please Him. But how could this forced strength actually interfere with genuine dependence on God?

We often try to keep our emotional pain hidden, but sometimes our feelings overwhelm us. If this happens, would it be better to break down in front of others or quickly excuse ourselves and escape to a place where we can be alone to deal with the situation? Explain your answer.

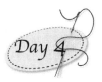

Cross Check

"Truth exists; only lies are invented."

George Braque

Though the military doctors at our new base were thorough and caring, numerous early treatments failed. Discouraged and longing for relief, I decided to locate the uro-gynecologist nearest our new home. Travel cost would be worth it, regardless of how far I had to go.

I called my previous uro-gynecologist for direction, never dreaming what God had planned for me.

The specialist was excited to hear from me. He'd just returned from a medical seminar in Chicago where he'd met a military doctor trained in uro-gynecology. And … the doctor was moving to our base in Texas in just a few weeks. What a mighty God we serve!

Upon the specialist's referral, the military doctor contacted me when he arrived, evaluated my test results, and suggested another surgery.

He was reluctant to reopen my incision, opting, instead, to perform less evasive surgery. He cautioned me ahead of time that the operation might not work. Nevertheless, I was devastated when I discovered I still couldn't void properly after surgery.

Once again, I fought recurring thoughts of unworthiness and condemnation for not being good enough to receive God's favor and healing.

In the Garden of Eden, Satan approached Eve with a lie—a direct contradiction to what God had said. "You will not surely die. For God knows that when you eat of it your eyes will be opened, and you will be like God, knowing good and evil" (Gen 3:4-5).

You know the story. Eve believed the devil and acted on her belief.

I wonder if Eve might have recognized Satan's deception if she had checked with God again before acting. "What, exactly, did You say about this tree?"

Old story—but relevant today because Satan is still in the business of deception. We are not worthy of God's love. God will never answer our prayers.

The words sound right, and our circumstances support them. Buying into the lies, we are caught in a vicious cycle. We become depressed . . . We feel guilty for being depressed . . . We become more depressed . . . We feel guiltier . . . and so on, until life is so jumbled we can't find God anywhere.

Eve accepted Satan's lie without question. We can learn from her mistake.

The Bible instructs us to examine our thoughts and line them up with Scripture. "Do your best to present yourself to God as one approved, a worker who does not need to be ashamed and who correctly handles the word of truth" (2 Timothy 2:15).

When we ask, the Holy Spirit will disclose our faulty thoughts. And as we practice correctly handling the Word of truth, we will learn to trap negative thoughts that threaten to bring us down before they do any damage.

So, rather than passively accepting lies, let's actively double-check our source. Let's ask, "Lord, what, exactly, did you say about loving me with unconditional, unfailing love?" And let's allow His answer to soak into our spirits with truth and healing.

> "But when He, the Spirit of truth, comes,
> He will guide you into all the truth."
>
> John 16:13a

Writing from the Heart
Healing...from the Inside Out

God brought the very type of doctor I needed to my new home. How has God blessed you in a time of transition?

What is the difference between conviction and condemnation? How can you keep them separate in your life?

Read the conversation in Luke 4:1-13. How does Jesus respond when tempted? How could we follow Christ's example in this way?

The Problem with Peace

"The weaker we feel, the harder we lean. And the harder we lean, the stronger we grow.

J. J. Packer

I couldn't believe it—a fourth surgery would be necessary somewhere down the road. After I healed from the third. The doctor explained that the surgery would be extremely risky because of the massive amount of scar tissue inside me.

I'd been raised to believe that Christians should have peace at all times. Surely, if I did enough of the God-things—praying, reading my Bible, attending church, etc., the anxiety would go away. But it didn't.

As I prayed about this, I remembered Romans 8:1. "There is now no condemnation for those who are in Christ Jesus." Conviction, yes. A deep, heart-felt remorse and desire to change. That is the leading of the Holy Spirit. But condemnation will never come from God, and when we blindly allow ourselves to walk in it, we are choosing a dangerous path.

As I grieved over not being good enough for God or achieving what He desired in my life, I was angry with myself for failing in my own power and strength. Why couldn't I do it? I wanted to. Why wasn't that enough?

But God never asked me to make myself into anything. He intended to do the work. Perfect work. Not vain attempts on my part to mimic what only He could accomplish.

In John 14:27, Jesus said, "Peace I leave with you; my peace I give you. I do not give to you as the world gives. Do not let your hearts be troubled and do not be afraid."

Peace from above. Sure, there will still be times when our hearts are troubled and we are afraid. Times when we wonder if we will ever again enjoy lasting peace in our hearts. It's in these times that we must turn to Christ. "For He Himself is our peace" (Ephesians 2:14a).

God desires honesty. He knows our thoughts and feelings. Our doubts and fears. And sometimes, He allows pain in our lives to wake us up. To alert us to the enemy's attacks on our minds. Our thought lives.

God is aware of that which seeks to destroy us from within, and He wants to free us from bondage to faulty thinking.

What is our responsibility in obtaining this peace from above? Quite simple, actually—we must seek Jesus. Years ago there was a popular bumper sticker that read: Know Jesus—Know Peace. No Jesus—No Peace. So very true.

We must deal with our feelings as they surface and ask the Holy Spirit to reveal our underlying thought processes. Why do we feel the way we do? What does the Bible say to support or contradict our thoughts? How can we purposely determine to change any incorrect thinking?

We should pray, "Search me, God, and know my heart; test me and know my anxious thoughts" (Psalm 139:23). And He will do just that.

As we surrender to God's care, listen to His voice, and obey His leading, God will renew our hearts and minds and change us into His image. From glory to glory.

> "Do not conform to the pattern of this world, but be transformed by the renewing of your mind."
>
> Romans 12:2a

Writing from the Heart
Healing...from the Inside Out

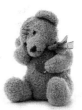

According to 1 Corinthians 13, love is to be patient and kind. It is not easily angered and keeps no record of wrongs. Why is it important that you apply these attributes to yourself as well as others?

Are there areas in your life in which you need to forgive yourself? Give yourself mercy?

Is it possible to love your neighbor appropriately if you don't love yourself?

Week 7:

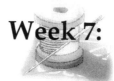

Chain-Stitched Circle of Friendship

"The greatest healing therapy is friendship and love."

Hubert H. Humphrey

Friends don't always know the best approach when talking about our pain. In fact, some get very nervous or, perhaps, avoid the subject altogether. I knew this, so I wasn't totally shocked at my pastors' behavior when they visited me in the hospital.

When they arrived, the youth pastor barely said hello before he scurried to the window, his eyes fixed on the parking lot below. "Hmm," I thought. "He'll have to get better at hospital visits."

Then Pastor started acting weird—talking about ninety miles an hour. Well, that wasn't really all that weird for Pastor. But he didn't blink. I mean, not the whole time he talked to me. He was like a rambling machine.

"Good grief," I thought. "I've got to talk to the church board. This just won't do. He is really making me feel uncomfortable."

Shortly, a close friend dropped by. As soon as she stepped in the door, the pastors said their goodbyes and vanished.

"Wow!" I said. "Pastor is really acting strange today."

"I wonder why," she pondered. "Got any idea?"

"No, I sure don't," I answered.

"Well, look down."

I was hooked up to an E.K.G. machine, dressed in v-neck pajamas that snapped up the front. The monitor's battery pack was tucked in the pocket of the shirt. Unfortunately, the weight of the pack had pulled the front of my shirt to the side, leaving you know what hanging out the front opening.

Poor pastors. Needless to say, I didn't mention the incident to the board—a bit of mercy seemed appropriate.

Living with pain is a lonely adventure. We long for a shoulder to lean on in the darkness of the night when tears fall in secret. But accepting help isn't always easy.

God knows what we hold inside. He sees through the masks we wear to disguise our pain and the walls we build to keep others out. He longs to help us. But sometimes, He has to wait until we are ready to accept help.

Edwin Cole said, "You don't drown by falling in the water; you drown by staying there."

Too often, when God reaches out His hand, we react like a drowning child who thrashes about wildly, actually hindering any attempts to save her. And like this victim, we will sink unless we acknowledge that we cannot help ourselves, stop struggling, and submit completely to the strength and direction of the One trying to save us.

In this week's lessons, we'll talk about pretending—the masks we wear to convince others we are doing fine. Maybe even to convince ourselves.

Friends want to help, but we hesitate to open up to them because we're not sure they could ever understand our struggle. But what if we took time to show our friends just what we need?

Finally, as we discuss how suffering without hope leads to depression and a desire to give up, we'll consider the possibility of getting *real* with others. With ourselves. And with God.

Will the Real Me Ever Stand Up?

"Until you have given up your self to Him you
will not have a real self."

C. S. Lewis

I was just a child, but I still remember going to sleep at night listening to "See the Funny Little Clown" by Bobby Goldsboro. Though the little clown was laughing on the outside, there was a tear in his eye. No one knew he was crying. No one knew he was dying—on the inside.

Six months had passed since my sister died in an automobile accident. Life seemed to have returned to normal. But then, what is normal?

Is it pretending you're doing fine, even though the ache within you feels like it's about to burn a hole through your heart? Is it laughing at jokes and making small talk to spare others the discomfort of having to respond to your pain? Is it being careful not to mention what is really on your mind twenty-four hours a day?

As I healed from my third surgery, I stayed close to home. *Pretending* took too much energy, and I was afraid I would break down emotionally. Friends wouldn't have minded, but I was embarrassed that this situation had gone on for so long. I felt guilty attracting attention *again.*

With time, a scab formed around my pain. Others saw me returning to everyday activities and assumed I was healing within. The scab, however, thickened and became more difficult to penetrate. I could no longer get to the pain. I could no longer cry to release the despair and sadness that accompanied me every second of my life.

You see, there's a reason I still remember the words to the song, even after fifty years. I've lived the role of the funny little clown—a smile on my face, despite the concealed pain I held inside.

The inner turmoil that accompanies chronic pain often threatens to overpower and control us. At times, it's nearly impossible to hold back tears, while everything seems to be going fine for everyone else. No one knows. No one has any idea that we are still crying into the wee hours of the morning. No one realizes that our smiles are so shallow.

We play the game. We continue to continue. All the while, we long for someone to help us through.

God knows us so well. He sees us crying on the inside, even when we're laughing on the outside. He's our best friend, never distracted or too busy. He remembers what we tell Him and never ridicules or condemns us. Just continues to hold and love us.

As we spend time with Him, our confusion will gradually turn to peace, our discouragement to hope, and our feebleness to strength.

The *real me* can then stand up, for it is not me, but Christ in me.

We can join the apostle Paul, proclaiming, "I have been crucified with Christ and I no longer live, but Christ lives in me. The life I live in the body, I live by faith in the Son of God, who loved me and gave Himself for me" (Galatians 2:20).

"Nothing in all creation is hidden from God's sight."
Hebrews 4:13a

Writing from the Heart
Healing...from the Inside Out

Who is the *real* you? Setting all pretenses aside, introduce yourself on paper. Include strengths and flaws.

How did your childhood experiences influence who you are today?

How might others describe you differently than you describe yourself? How do you feel about the difference? What would be a good reason for these two descriptions to be closely matched?

Day 2

The Bottom is a Long Way Down.
I Know ... I Hit It.

"God whispers to us in our pleasures, speaks in our
conscience, but shouts in our pains; it is His
megaphone to rouse a deaf world."

C.S. Lewis

One morning I woke to excruciating pain. Nonetheless, I
dressed for work, mumbling, "Life must go on. I can't stay
home forever."

By the time I arrived at school, however, I couldn't even
stand.

As friends helped prepare for a substitute, I felt numb and
disoriented. "I don't care," I answered when they asked me
questions. "I just don't want to live anymore."

I'd hit bottom. I went home and cried uncontrollably for over
an hour. Then I began to talk to Jesus. "I don't know how I
should be feeling, but this is where I'm at. I can't be strong any
more. The devil is winning. I'm sinking into a dark black hole,
and I can't get out."

I fell asleep, and when I woke, I felt physically refreshed, as if
I'd slept for days. The Lord spoke softly to my spirit. "The
trial is going to end. One does eventually get through the
deep waters—there is another side. I'm not causing the pain,
but I will bring something good from it."

I wanted to remember the pain. The discouragement and hopelessness. Some day, I wanted to be able to minister with genuine empathy to others who hurt like I did. So I recorded my feelings.

Suffering without hope leads to depression, to a desire to give up, to end it all. I wouldn't do anything because I love God and my family, and I know it would be wrong. But I can't keep the ideas from coming to my head. My strength is gone, and it's so hard to live. People don't want to be around someone who constantly talks about her problems, so I just cover up. I act fine. No one knows, except for just a few.

When someone asks how I'm doing, I say fine. If they change the subject and go on to something else, I conclude that they don't really care—that I can't confide in them. And it hurts. I want them to know that I'm really not fine, and I want them to be concerned enough to probe. I only confide in those who say they really want to know. That kind of persistent love gets to me—the thought that someone really does care about me.

Chronic pain warped my thoughts. But however distorted, my perceptions were reality to me. What I wanted more than anything else, I refused to ask for. A listening ear. A shoulder to cry on. Understanding, intense prayer. *Praying through*, as we used to say. Talking to God until the burden lifts and peace takes its place.

We can't stay home forever. We have to press on, pain or no pain. But we don't have to do it alone. Others are hurting all around us. Probably saying they're *fine*.

Suppose we choose to get real. Purpose to carry each other's burdens. Spend time together, honestly sharing our hearts. Crying. Praying. Loving each other—as Christ would do if He were here. Because He is.

"Therefore confess your sins to each other and pray for each other so that you may be healed. The prayer of a righteous person is powerful and effective."

James 5:16

Writing from the Heart

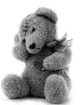

Healing...from the Inside Out

What keeps you from confiding in and asking for the help of others?

How could admitting your pain and distress actually help someone else?

How could trying to *appear* strong and happy actually bring you closer to the dark, black hole of depression?

My Bandage Isn't Sticking

"You don't realize Jesus is all you need
until Jesus is all you have."

Tim Keller

One morning, a few months after we moved to Texas, I wrote God a letter.

Today is Sunday, and a big part of me is excited about church. But another part is afraid my mask will crumble. The music. The message. Your Holy Spirit penetrating the protective shell I try so hard to hide behind. Prayer times are scary. My bandage isn't sticking as well—there's too much seepage, and I can't control it anymore.

The Holy Spirit stirs within me and I want to run. A couple of times I've relented and gone forward to the altar, crying out to You in my distress. You soothed my soul as I opened my deepest self to you. But when it was time to leave, I was emotionally wide open—exposed and vulnerable to others who weren't experiencing emotional upheaval at the time. Conversation was meant to be light as folks asked how things were going.

It's so hard to simply smile and answer, "Fine." My heart longs for someone to hold me, to really care how it's going. But that doesn't happen on the way out of church.

There's so much locked inside of me. I'm good at pretending everything's fine, but it's getting to me. I'm cracking. Pain is beginning to creep out—to surface when I least expect it. I'm losing control. There are times when I can't push the pain back. The tears come and I can't stop them.

This person within my person is screaming to be acknowledged and set free. Oh, Father, what can I do?

I went to church that morning, and God revealed Himself to me in a special way. When I got home, I finished my letter with a lighter heart.

Thank You, Lord, for Your love today. As I stood in Your presence, I came to You as a little child. As I sat on Your lap and leaned against Your chest, You held me gently. You wiped my tears and comforted me.

Then You showed me I need to come to You often as my heart mends. That as I heal emotionally, my body and soul can withstand some pressure, but that if I don't return for Your touch, the cracks will separate again. Fresh pain will surface as new flesh is ripped open. Scarring will develop and healing will be impeded.

I need Your arms around me like a vice, to hold me together.

What a beautiful thought. The arms of Jesus holding His broken child together while His healing power restores and renews. His loving arms providing the strength and refuge we so desperately seek and need.

For various reasons, many of us don't have a strong support system. Family members and friends, though gentle and kind, don't understand our physical and emotional condition.

But God does. He sees what others cannot and promises in Psalm 139 to "hem us in." To encircle us with His presence and bind our hearts as we heal—from the inside out.

"He heals the brokenhearted and binds up their wounds."

Psalm 147:3

Writing from the Heart
Healing...from the Inside Out

What is the difference between being friendly and being a friend? Could this affect our ability to be honest with others?

So often, when we censor our own thoughts and feelings, we avoid dealing honestly with them. Ask God to reveal the depths of your heart and write about what He shows you without trying to apologize for or justify what you see. Just get it down on paper.

A bandage can temporarily fix a wound. But true healing will only come when the wound is opened, cleansed, and treated. Then the bandage protects the work that has been done until the area is ready to be exposed without risk of reinfection. How could this apply to your emotional life?

Day 4

What Do I Need?

> "If we have no peace, it is because we have
> forgotten that we belong to each other."
>
> Mother Teresa

Throughout this journey, one thing remained constant: God's grace. Each time I approached the Lord with despair and uncertainty, He responded with assurance—mercy, to look beyond my belief, and grace, to give me the hope I desperately needed. God helped me through so many things.

At one point, I came upon 2 Corinthians 1:3-4. "Praise be to the God and Father of our Lord Jesus Christ, the Father of compassion and the God of all comfort, who comforts us in all our troubles, so that we can comfort those in any trouble with the comfort we ourselves receive from God."

So many times, we see others in pain, and we don't know how to respond. I wanted to remember how I felt so that I could, one day, minister to others in similar pain. I wrote:

What do I need? I need to know you care. I need to know that you're not tired of hearing about my problems because this has gone on for a long time. I need to know that you don't think I have sin in my life, or not enough faith, because I can't handle condemnation right now. I'm ready to break.

It really hurts for someone to ask how I am and not follow through. And then, there are those friends who cared so much at first. I trusted them and relied on their prayers and their calls, and now, they never ask.

But I still need help. I'm sorry this is going on so long. Please keep loving me. Please let me know you're still praying. I'm ready to crack.

Of course, I never voiced these feelings. I just assumed my friends didn't know how to minister to me. But it hurt. Why couldn't they see what I needed? Why couldn't God show them?

I could have—probably should have—enlightened my friends. So often, they asked, "What can we do?"

Why *did* I hold back?

Why do we so often pretend to be something we're not? Why do we insist on blocking God's healing love that flows through the body of Christ?

For some, it might involve pride. We're used to being overcomers. Self-sufficient. We don't want others to see weakness in us.

Or maybe we believe we need to be strong for those who depend on us for stability and direction. That if we show our weakness, we'll let them down. Maybe even cause them to stumble in their Christian walk.

For me, it was about a lack of self worth. I didn't want to bother others or waste their time. Didn't want to selfishly solicit attention others might need more than I did.

Distorted thinking, sad as it is. Especially if we transfer it to our concept of God's love.

Walking in truth with others takes courage. Faith that God will give us words to say. That He will prepare others' hearts to understand as we share our deepest hurts and needs. That God will bond us together in His love.

"Finally, all of you, be like-minded, be sympathetic, love one another, be compassionate and humble."

1 Peter 3:8

Writing from the Heart

Healing...from the Inside Out

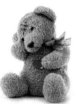

Do you think we ought to help our friends understand how they can help us?

Why would you want a friend to be that honest with you?

What do you need right now? Can you think of someone else to whom you could be that listening ear and shoulder to cry on?

Jesus Looked at Him and Loved Him

*"We cannot always trace God's hand, but
we can always trust God's heart."*

Charles Spurgeon

Let me tell you about Tyler, a shy little six-year-old with huge brown eyes and a priceless smile. One day as we were doing math, I wandered through the room, watching to be sure each student was doing the work correctly. "Need some help, buddy?" I asked.

"No, thanks. I'm okay," Tyler answered with a wide smile.

But as I stepped away and glanced back, I saw that Tyler had only three problems finished, while many of the other students had already completed the entire assignment. I looked more closely. The first two of Tyler's problems were wrong and the third was nothing but a smudged hole where he had erased and erased and erased. That poor little guy must have been so frustrated. So confused and embarrassed. Yet he assured me that he was fine. He wanted to please me.

Talk about melting. I wanted to hug him. Gently, I patted Tyler on the shoulder and told him I appreciated his hard work. Then I pulled out a fresh sheet of paper and solved the problem for him as he watched. My heart soared as he sat up straight and tackled number four with renewed strength and confidence. As he completed his work, I checked on Tyler often, encouraging and supporting him when necessary.

Suddenly, I pictured Jesus by my side, watching to be sure *I* was truly okay—that I had grasped what He set before me for that day.

But, He also showed me that I have a choice to make. I can say, "I'm okay, Lord," and cover my frustrations, or I can raise my hand and ask for His help.

We have been in Tyler's place too often. Without realizing it, we rely on our own strength and then feel bad about disappointing the Lord when we fail.

Mark 10:17-21 tells of a young man who also tried hard to do things right. Running to Jesus, he asked, "Good teacher, what must I do to inherit eternal life?"

Jesus instructed him to obey His commandments, and the young man replied, "Teacher, all these I have kept since I was a boy."

Hearing and understanding, "Jesus looked at him and loved him." I love that part! Jesus sees and loves our efforts—as clumsy as they might be.

Just as I shielded my students from frustration, God watches over us. He holds the answers we need, but first He must convince us that it is okay to need help. Too often, we wear ourselves out trying to continue as if life is fine when, just like little Tyler, we need to remember that it is not our successful performance that pleases God, but our willingness to seek His help.

If we will but turn to God, allowing Him to be our strength and guide, He will pull out a fresh sheet of paper and show us the way, standing by our side to encourage and support us. He will stay nearby forever, ready to help whenever we ask.

"For the eyes of the Lord range throughout the earth to strengthen those whose hearts are fully committed to Him."

2 Chronicles 16:9a

Writing from the Heart

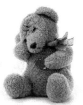

Healing...from the Inside Out

How do you get caught up in the performance trap? Do you find yourself believing that the more you read your Bible, pray, and serve the Lord, the more pleased He is with you?

We know that God looks at the heart, not the outward appearance. Does that mean He doesn't care about our behavior or appearance at all? What does the Bible say about this in Romans 13:12-14 and Colossians 3:12-17?

What can you do, personally, to remind yourself that God is standing by your side, ready to encourage you, show you how to solve your problems, and offer you a fresh start every moment of your life?

. . . the Rest of the Story

As I walked through this journey to health, I found the arms of Jesus always extended and ready to hold me. I learned to easily recognize the strong voice of the Holy Spirit speaking gently over the roar of the storm.

I took notes. I wanted to remember the pain, the restoring touch of my Father's hand, and the strength of His arms, so I could pray fervently for others in the future. I wanted to remember so I could tell others what God had done for me.

As I jotted down my deepest feelings on the corners of church bulletins, on the back of grocery lists, and on any sort of paper available at the moment I needed it, the Lord spoke clearly to me, planting the seed in my heart to write this book.

He said, "I want others to discover the peace you've discovered as you spent time with Me, listening to My gentle voice. I want them to see how your burdens were lifted as you surrendered your fears, doubts, guilt, and confusion to Me and allowed Me to fill that void with My love and assurance. I want others to cry as you cried and rejoice as you rejoiced. I want them to know Me through you. Will you do that for Me?"

"Yes, Lord. I will."

130

I have shared my heart. My fourth surgery was successful. The doctor removed the stitches from the original surgery so that my bladder returned to a proper tilt, and I was able to void consistently and completely. Recovery took a few weeks, but I was free of infection and constant muscle spasms. Free of non-stop pain.

Through the years since these surgeries, however, I've continued to suffer with the chronic pain of arthritis, degenerative discs in my back, and frequent migraines. But as I deal with this continuous, almost daily, pain and occasionally begin to question God's love, the Holy Spirit brings the lessons in this book to my mind. And I am able to rest in God, knowing that He didn't call me to understand. He called me to trust Him, and I do.

Many would have given up on God through all of this. I am occasionally tempted. But each time I am at my lowest, He gives me His Highest.

"I remain confident of this: I will see the goodness of the Lord in the land of the living. Wait for the Lord; be strong and take heart and wait for the Lord."

Psalm 24:17

53118219R00080

Made in the USA
Middletown, DE
25 November 2017